China's Health Silk Road

In memory of my primary school (启蒙) teachers
Mr Luk, who thought so highly of my Chinese calligraphy
and
Madam Fung, who made the learning of classical Chinese so
much fun.

China's Health Silk Road

Vaccine Diplomacy and Health Governance

Gerald Chan

*Professor Emeritus of Politics and International Relations,
School of Social Sciences, University of Auckland, New Zealand*

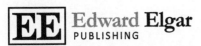

Edward Elgar
PUBLISHING

Cheltenham, UK • Northampton, MA, USA

Published by
Edward Elgar Publishing Limited
The Lypiatts
15 Lansdown Road
Cheltenham
Glos GL50 2JA
UK

Edward Elgar Publishing, Inc.
William Pratt House
9 Dewey Court
Northampton
Massachusetts 01060
USA

A catalogue record for this book
is available from the British Library

Library of Congress Control Number: 2023924652

This book is available electronically in the **Elgar**online
Political Science and Public Policy subject collection
http://dx.doi.org/10.4337/9781035320202

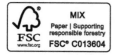

ISBN 978 1 0353 2019 6 (cased)
ISBN 978 1 0353 2020 2 (eBook)

Printed and bound by CPI Group (UK) Ltd, Croydon, CR0 4YY

Contents

Figures

Tables

Preface and acknowledgements

The year 2023 marks the tenth anniversary of the Belt and Road Initiative (BRI) and the fourth anniversary of the outbreak of Covid-19 in Wuhan.

I started to study China's One Belt One Road (OBOR) in 2015, as the Belt and Road Initiative was then commonly known. To the native Chinese and in the term that they use, the initiative is still known as 一带一路, or One Belt One Road, up to this day. Two things caught my imagination at that time: one was the fast development of China's high-speed rail system; the other was the little-known organisation called the Asian Infrastructure Investment Bank. It was founded in 2015 and started to extend its first batch of loans in 2016. Now it is a well-known institution in the global financial market and the development community.

This initial study of mine about OBOR resulted in a trilogy published by Edward Elgar Publishing, UK:

1. *Understanding China's new diplomacy: silk roads and bullet trains* (2018).
2. *China's maritime Silk Road: advancing global development?* (2020).
3. *China's digital Silk Road: setting standards, powering growth* (2022).

This book here would complete a quartet.

The rise of China has long become a cliché, but this cliché still floats around these days, for some tangible reasons. In April 2022 the World Bank adjusted the global economic growth for the year from 4.1 per cent to 3.2 per cent as a result of the war in Ukraine.[1] According to the IMF, the growth for 2022 was 3.4 per cent, based on which the forecast for 2023 was 2.8 per cent before settling at 3.0 per cent in 2024.[2] China's growth in the first quarter of 2022 registered a respectable 4.8 per cent, a rise over the same quarter in the previous year, followed by 0.4 per cent, 3.9 per cent and 2.9 per cent in the subsequent quarters.[3] Forecasts for China's growth in 2023 crowded around 5.5 per cent as of August 2023.[4]

While ploughing through my third book on China's Belt and Road dealing with the digital dimension, around mid-2021, I was toying with the idea of possibly following up with a fourth volume – perhaps on the topic of the Health Silk Road. At first, I was a bit hesitant, not sure whether there would be sufficient material out there to draw on to make up a reasonably good-sized manuscript, until the long-term effect of the Covid-19 pandemic became evident. So I decided to do some preliminary reading and exploration. One idea led to another, and the end result is this book.

Among other things, the book provides a Chinese perspective on Sino–US relations, especially in dealing with the politics of health (Chapter 7).

During the course of research and writing, I have benefited from many discussions with friends and colleagues, discussions that flowed from the talks that I gave on some aspects of the book:

1. A talk titled 'Can China's Billionaires Help To Save the Covid World?' at my home institution, the University of Auckland, on 23 November 2022;
2. A webinar on 'Can China's Billionaires Help To Save the World from Pandemics?' at Tokyo International University on 26 April 2023; and
3. A talk on 'Patient Rights vs Patent Rights: A Cruel Choice for China?' at the Taipei School of Economics and Political Science, Hsinchu, Taiwan, on 9 May 2023.

Along the solitary path of research, sometimes all by myself, I have accumulated a lot of debt to a lot of people. I am particularly grateful to my colleagues in Auckland for years of being together in teaching and research. I have learned handsomely from them, more than they might realise. One of them was amazed that I would embark on such an 'ambitious' project as the Health Silk Road. My Head of the School of Social Sciences, Associate Professor Katharine Smits, has been exceptionally supportive in more ways than one.

I am also grateful to the four reviewers who took time to go through my book proposal and offered their professional opinions. I think I have taken in most of their ideas. Any shortcomings that remain in the book are mine alone.

I couldn't forget how I have cherished my long association with Dr Pak K. Lee of the University of Kent, UK, and Dr Lai-Ha Chan of the University of Technology Sydney, for their friendship, encouragement and professional help. We all share our joy and tribulations in our investigation into China's health governance in our book *China Engages Global Governance* (2012).[5] That joint project has inevitably sowed the seed for this book.

My family of four were able to get together for a very happy reunion in Hong Kong in the (northern) summer of 2023. For the bigger, extended Chan family in Hong Kong, it was particularly meaningful, as it was a reunion after a lapse of three Covid years. All this was made possible thanks to a visiting professorship so kindly offered me by the Chinese University of Hong Kong during July, where I did my final revision of this book manuscript using the library collections in the Universities Service Centre and the Main University

Library. The Institute of Chinese Studies at the same University provided me with office and IT facilities, for which I remain truly grateful.

Gerald Chan
Stonefields, Auckland

Note: All currencies cited in this book are in US dollars unless otherwise specified. Chinese, Japanese, Korean, and Vietnamese names are presented with surname/family name first, followed by given name(s).

NOTES

1.   BBC World News, 19 April 2022.
2.   See https:// www .imf .org/ en/ Publications/ WEO #: ~: text = Description %3A %20The%20baseline%20forecast%20is,to%201.3%20percent%20in%202023 (accessed 19 June 2023).
3.   See https://www.statista.com/statistics/271769/quarterly-gross-domestic-product -gdp-growth-rate-in-china/ (accessed 20 June 2023).
4.   For example, Standard Chartered's forecast was 5.4 per cent (*Ming bao*, Hong Kong, 19 July 2023, p. B3).
5.   Gerald Chan, Pak K. Lee, and Lai-Ha Chan, *China engages global governance: a new world order in the making?* (London and New York: Routledge, 2012).

Abbreviations

ADB	Asian Development Bank
AI	artificial intelligence
AIIB	Asian Infrastructure Investment Bank
APEC	Asia-Pacific Economic Cooperation
APIs	active pharmaceutical ingredients
ASEAN	Association of Southeast Asian Nations
AUKUS	Australia, UK, US
BRI	Belt and Road Initiative
BRICS	Brazil, Russia, India, China, South Africa
CDC	Center for Disease Control and Prevention
CIA	Central Intelligence Agency
CSIS	Center for Strategic and International Studies
EU	European Union
GAVI	Global Alliance for Vaccines and Immunisation
GCI	Global Civilisation Initiative
GDI	Global Development Initiative
GDP	Gross Domestic Product
GSI	Global Security Initiative
HSR	Health Silk Road
ICD	International Classification of Diseases
IMF	International Monetary Fund
IP	intellectual property
IPE	international political economy
ISO	International Organisation for Standardisation
IT	information technology
KSMs	key starting materials
MERICS	Mercator Institute for China Studies

MIIT	Ministry of Industry and Information Technology
mRNA	messenger ribonucleic acid
NDRC	National Development and Reform Commission
OECD	Organisation for Economic and Cooperation Development
PCT	Patent Cooperation Treaty
PLA	People's Liberation Army
PRC	People's Republic of China
R&D	Research and development
RMB	Renminbi (Chinese currency, or yuan)
SAC	Standardisation Administration of China
SCO	Shanghai Cooperation Organisation
SOEs	State-owned enterprises
T&CM	Traditional and complementary medicine
TCM	Traditional Chinese medicine
TRIPS	Trade-Related Aspects of Intellectual Property Rights
UK	United Kingdom
UN	United Nations
UNCTAD	United Nations Conference on Trade and Development
UNDP	United Nations Development Programme
UNESCO	United Nations Educational, Scientific and Cultural Organisation
UNSDGs	United Nations Sustainable Development Goals
US	United States
WHO	World Health Organisation
WIPO	World Intellectual Property Organisation
WTO	World Trade Organisation

1. Introduction to *China's Health Silk Road*

Health is wealth! The Covid-19 pandemic has clearly brought home the importance of keeping well and staying safe. China's Health Silk Road (HSR), which began as a relatively little-noticed component of the Belt and Road Initiative (BRI), has now become an attractive way for China to develop and promote its interests in the health sector. The country was not known for mass producing vaccines before the outbreak of the new coronavirus in late 2019, but two years later it had become the biggest exporter of Covid-19 vaccines in the world, under the flagship of its vaccine diplomacy. So, what is this vaccine diplomacy? How has it come about?

China's vaccine diplomacy poses a puzzle: What is the country's stand in the debate that has been raging fiercely for quite some time between those who advocate the importance of maintaining the existing patent-rights system covering medicines and those who champion the goal of asserting the rights of patients to gain access to affordable life-saving drugs? Patient rights are particularly pertinent to the developing world where many people can ill afford to buy expensive drugs. China's stand in this debate is little noticed, in large part because it is a latecomer to the game. However, as the country rises to become a significant healthcare provider in the world, its position has become pivotal for global health governance. Does China's involvement in these two issues – vaccine diplomacy and the debates surrounding the conflict between patent rights and patient rights – make any serious difference to the way global health is governed? If so, to what extent?

China aspires to become a global leader in the bio-pharmaceutical industry. This aspiration was made clear in 'Made in China 2025', a programme adopted in 2015 with the aim of nurturing ten critical technologies to become world leaders within ten years. Apart from biomedicine, others include high-speed rail, maritime engineering, the aerospace industry, information technology, robotic science, and so on. Can China turn itself into the pharmaceutical factory of the world? If it can, how will it affect the existing architecture of global health? In what way will the poor in the Global South benefit from China's HSR – now becoming a catchphrase for the country's health diplomacy?

Despite China's increasing prominence in the global public health sector, there is as yet little or no book-length treatment in the area. This book tries to fill this gap, and also a gap in my study of China's BRI. I have written three books relating to the BRI: the first traces the overland Silk Road and focuses on the development of high-speed rail (published in 2018)[1]; the second charts the maritime Silk Road (2020)[2]; and the third explores the digital Silk Road (2022).[3] This book on the health component forms a fourth volume in the series.

Domestically, the HSR has become a catalyst for promoting the well-being of the country's populace. Externally, it has the potential to benefit people abroad, especially those in the Global South. The large and dense population in the eastern part of the country and the close contacts between humans and animals have meant that viruses have a great chance to jump from animals to humans (and vice versa).[4] China has become a hotbed for epidemics,[5] something the country and its people have grown somewhat used to in crowded living and working conditions. However, the ability to deal effectively with viruses and to control their spread is of great concern, not only to China but also to the world at large, as viruses can spread with no respect for geographic boundary or political sovereignty.

The outbreak of Covid-19 has dramatically changed the flow of the global supply of vaccines. The virus has thrust China to the forefront of the spread and control of the pandemic. Is the country on course to become a new superpower in medical supplies, as it aspires to do? What have the United States (US) and the European Union (EU) done to face this challenge from China? This book tracks the rise of China's vaccine diplomacy. It locates the country's position in the debates between patent rights and patient rights, between big pharmaceutical companies who hold the world's major patents of drugs and the poor people around the world who struggle to gain access to life-saving medicines. China is caught between a rock and a hard place: on the one hand, it has declared Covid-19 vaccines to be global public goods, aiming to ease their availability to all; on the other, it is quickly becoming a large owner of patents itself, holding potentially increased power and influence over the flow of drugs. So, will the HSR lead to better healthcare for all?

This introductory chapter spells out the objectives of the book. It then establishes what the HSR is, including its origins and development. This is followed by a brief introduction to the book's approach. I use the term *geo-developmentalism* as the guide, an idea that I have developed over the past few years, which serves as a theoretical lens for studying the HSR. The chapter concludes by laying out the plan of the book with brief overviews of subsequent chapters.

THE AIM OF THIS BOOK

This book aims to enhance our understanding of what China has accomplished and what the country plans to contribute towards improving global public health. It uses China's HSR as a vehicle to assist us in this process. China's reaching out to the global health system proceeds as the country continues to rise in economic and political power. In examining China's efforts, the book helps unpack some of the complexities surrounding the working of the global public health system which resulted from the outbreak of Covid-19 and its ravaging of the world.

In reviewing China's drive to build its HSR, the book provides a greater understanding of China's new diplomacy. What is the HSR? What are its origins? How has it developed? How does it relate to the country's BRI, especially the digital Silk Road? This is where technology meets health, generating new possibilities for dealing with increasing demands for better healthcare and for improving the well-being of citizens under economic and social constraints.

This book contends that China has started to make a substantial contribution towards helping other countries deal with health problems, especially those countries in the Global South, as highlighted during the spread of the Covid-19 pandemic. It also argues that the country favours the rights of patients to life-saving drugs over the rights of patents held by pharmaceutical companies covering those drugs. China's actions have helped narrow the gap in the provision of healthcare that exists among the world's rich and poor countries. From a larger perspective, it can be seen that they have helped reduce the imbalance and inequity in wealth distribution.

WHAT IS THE HEALTH SILK ROAD?

The term 'Health Silk Road' is the new designation for China's foreign medical assistance programme. As such, it has a history dating back to the 1960s when China started to provide aid to developing countries around the world, especially in Africa. Medical aid has remained a significant part of the country's foreign aid. China's official paper explaining the new Silk Road in 2015 highlighted health cooperation with other countries. In June 2016 President Xi Jinping delivered a speech at the Legislative Chamber of the Uzbek Supreme Assembly in Tashkent in which he stressed the importance of building a 'green, healthy, intelligent and peaceful Silk Road'.[6] The name 'Health Silk Road' was used by President Xi in his video address to the G20 Global Health Summit in Rome in May 2021 and in his telephone conversation with Italian Prime Minister Giuseppe Conte in March 2020. The HSR has gained media attention due largely to the outbreak of the new coronavirus, Covid-19. It has made substantial contributions to strengthen Chinese foreign policy under the broad umbrella of the BRI launched in 2013.

The HSR is more than just aid. It also involves trade and industry, and hence development in the long run. The other major components of the BRI, such as the land-based economic belt and the maritime Silk Road, also carry some elements of aid, but they largely include trade, investments, infrastructure construction, and development in nature. Again, like the land-based and maritime Silk Roads, many of the infrastructure projects undertaken along the HSR began well before 2013, the official starting year of the BRI.

Different people have different ideas about what constitutes the HSR. In the main, it is China's global health policy. It is so called probably because it is more easily recollected as a catchphrase. So it would be easier to publicise, especially when riding on the goodwill (infamous to some critics) generated by the BRI, as China's flagship foreign policy.

As indicated earlier, the idea of the HSR was derived from a reference to the health issues in an official document published in 2015 titled 'Vision and Action on Jointly Building the Silk Road Economic Belt and the 21st Century Maritime Silk Road'. The document lays out five types of connections to link various parts of the world through infrastructure building: policy coordination, physical infrastructure, financial cooperation, trade, and people-to-people contacts. Under the people-to-people contacts, the document stresses, among other things, health connections in the following way[7]:

> We should strengthen cooperation with neighbouring countries on epidemic information sharing, the exchange of prevention and treatment technologies and the training of medical professionals, and improve our capability to jointly address public health emergencies. We will provide medical assistance and emergency medical aid to relevant countries, and carry out practical cooperation in maternal and child health, disability rehabilitation, and major infectious diseases including AIDS, tuberculosis, and malaria. We will also expand cooperation on traditional medicine.

THE ORIGINS AND DEVELOPMENT OF THE HEALTH SILK ROAD

Many China watchers have picked 2015 as the starting year of the HSR because reference was made to it then as part of China's BRI. This reference can be found in the 'Vision and Action' policy paper of March 2015 mentioned above. The year appears somewhat arbitrary because some Chinese commentators have pointed out that the HSR was officially launched in 2016.[8] In any case, since March 2015, a number of major developments have been made, marking significant progress in the building of the HSR. These include[9]:

- The release in October 2015 of a three-year plan to promote health exchanges and cooperation among BRI countries by the Chinese National Health Commission.
- President Xi Jinping addressed the Uzbekistan Supreme Assembly in June 2016, calling for increased cooperation in infectious disease prevention

and information sharing, medical assistance, and traditional medicine development as a way to build the HSR.

- The issue of the 'Healthy China 2030' blueprint by the State Council in October 2016. This blueprint aims to raise China's health standards to match those found in developed countries by 2030. It also aims to meet the targets set by the United Nations 2030 Agenda for Sustainable Development, especially in the area of health and well-being.
- The signing of the China–World Health Organization (WHO) Country Cooperation Strategy (2016–2020) in Beijing in 2016.[10] This strategy focuses on cooperation in health policies, planning, technology, and human resources.
- The signing of a memorandum of understanding (MoU) with the WHO in January 2017 on the Implementation Plan on the Belt and Road Health Cooperation Mechanism, during President Xi's visit to the WHO in Geneva. This MoU aims to promote cooperation in health emergency response, prevention and treatment of infectious diseases, and traditional medicine among countries along the Belt and Road.[11]
- Following the first Belt and Road Forum for International Cooperation in August 2017, Beijing held a high-profile conference, bringing together senior health officials from 30 countries and representatives from some international health organisations including the WHO. A joint communiqué was issued to lay out a framework for promoting health cooperation and the HSR.
- Since then, China has organised numerous forums to discuss health issues, including the China–ASEAN Health Forum, the China–Central and Eastern European Countries Health Ministers Forum, and the China–Arab States Health Forum, among others.
- In a phone conversation between President Xi Jinping and Italian Prime Minister Giuseppe Conte on 16 March 2020, Xi said that China was 'ready to work with Italy to contribute to international cooperation on epidemic control and to the building of a "Health Silk Road"'.[12]

We will revisit some of these events in greater detail in the following chapters when they inform our analysis.

GEO-DEVELOPMENTALISM: THEORISING THE HEALTH SILK ROAD

The year 2023 marks the tenth anniversary of the BRI (known initially as One Belt, One Road, or *yidai yilu* 一带一路 when President Xi Jinping launched it in 2013) (See Appendix on a chronology of the BRI). Ten years on, the initiative has generated a large amount of empirical data covering numerous projects in many industrial sectors in a growing number of countries.[13] The number of countries that have signed Belt and Road cooperation documents has increased from an initial 34 to 151.[14] Wang Wen, the executive dean of the Chongyang Institute for Financial Studies at Renmin University in Beijing, pointed out that over 4000 investment projects worth $4 trillion have been launched under the BRI during its first decade.[15] In Africa, more than 10 000 km of roads, 6000 km of railways, and nearly 20 ports have been built.[16] In terms of trade, from 2013 to 2022, the total import and export volume per year between China and the Belt and Road countries increased from $1.04 trillion to $2.07 trillion, with an average annual growth rate of about 8 per cent.[17] And in terms of investments, China's non-financial direct investment in Belt and Road countries reached $182.2 billion from 2013 to 2022, accounting for about 20 per cent of the country's total overseas investment,[18] while two-way investments had topped $230 billion by the end of 2021.[19] The implementation of the BRI has generated a lot of responses from other countries: some are cooperative in nature while others are competitive or rivalrous.

So far, the theorising of the initiative has lagged far behind its practice, for understandable reasons such as academic interest, researchers' preference, and the complexity of the enterprise. Initial theorisation has largely been focused on mercantilism or neo-mercantilism. A group of scholars based in Singapore led by Shaun Lin, Naoko Shimazu, and James D. Sidaway have done some useful work to summarise the theorising efforts in the research community up to 2021.[20] They have put these efforts into four categories: geopolitics, geo-economics, Chinese exceptionalism, and Silk Road imaginary. Geopolitics and geo-economics can be seen as derivatives of neo-mercantilism. Chinese exceptionalism can be viewed as an approach similar to Chinese characteristics or Chinese uniqueness, which is fondly adopted by many China scholars, most of whom are based in mainland China. The Silk Road imaginary brings into the relevant body of knowledge some strong social constructivist elements to understand international relations and global political economy. In their efforts to draw implications of BRI theorising, Lin and his colleagues also try to look into the area of development studies to make new connections with existing development theories. This is done with a view to foster new insights, especially in the area of uneven development.

Other scholars have also tried to employ existing theories of international politics developed mainly in the West to study the BRI. In a book chapter titled 'Theorising the Belt and Road Initiative',[21] Jeremy Garlick uses such selective theories as Tang Shiping's social evolution paradigm, Robert Cox's neo-Gramscian hegemony, and Jonathan Holslag's offensive realism to explain the impact of the BRI.[22]

I myself have proposed a new way to look at the development of China's BRI. I put forward the idea of geo-developmentalism first in my book published in 2018 on the BRI. I have refined the idea over the years in my following two books, respectively on China's maritime Silk Road and its digital Silk Road. Here I continue to fine-tune and deploy geo-developmentalism as a theoretical lens to look at the working of the HSR.

I define geo-developmentalism as 'a China-initiated developmental trajectory of infrastructure building aimed at promoting mutual economic growth by increasing connections across the globe'. I have identified ten features of geo-developmentalism. Some of these features have seen their rise and fall in popularity in the media and in academic works, but all of them seem to have stayed intact as useful entry points to study the BRI. They have also proved to be useful for explaining the progress of the various Belt and Road projects and for assessing their viability and validity. A few of them have remained critical to understanding the BRI, China's flagship foreign policy. These include the win–win approach, the focus on infrastructure building, and the interaction between geo-economics and geopolitics. The building of the HSR in the Global South, especially in Africa, has provided valuable empirical evidence for testing the functionalities of these features (to be elaborated in Chapter 5).

The fact that many countries in the West have proposed their own initiatives to help build infrastructure in developing countries is a testimony of the market need of such projects for global development and the need to compete with China to build projects of better quality. Geo-developmentalism, although initiated by China, has been followed by others albeit in different forms and styles to fit into different political agendas. As such, China's influence in global governance, including the health sector, has a notable effect on the behaviour of others.

In contributing to global development, China is not only sticking to the promotion of the BRI. It has branched out to propose the Global Development Initiative to support the United Nations (UN) in achieving the Sustainable Development Goals (SDGs). More recently, the country has also proposed the Global Security Initiative and the Global Civilisation Initiative. We shall return to these new initiatives in Chapter 8.

THE PLAN OF THIS BOOK

This book consists of eight chapters. The first chapter – this one – is an introduction. The next one, Chapter 2, titled 'Building Silk Roads: Land, Sea, Digital, Health', sets the HSR against the context of the BRI. That initiative composes, in the main, the overland Silk Road, the maritime Silk Road, the digital Silk Road, and the HSR. The chapter brings these four components together to give a comprehensive picture of China's drive to develop, both domestically and globally. It argues that the digital component underpins the development of the others. They work together, however, in a holistic way,

forming a unique 'infrastructure of development' in contrast to the 'infrastructure of democracy' which has been developing over the past centuries in the
West. As a component working at a critical point in time, the HSR affects in
a major way the outcomes of the development of the other three. The Covid-19
pandemic is a case in point. Towards the end of the chapter we shall discuss
the development of telehealth in China, including internet hospitals – a new
venture at the forefront of medical innovation.

Chapter 3, titled 'The Global Structure of Public Health', sets out the global
context against which to examine the status and position of China's HSR. The
context canvasses the development of contemporary capitalism, a practice led
by the West, and its discourse on the rise of capitalism, imperialism, and neoliberalism. The chapter seeks to answer these questions: What is the structure
of the global health system? To what extent are China's health policies and
practices constrained or facilitated by this structure and by the international
order controlled largely by the West? The global health system is part and
parcel of this political-economic system. What are the avenues available
to China to pursue the protection of its health and national interests? This
chapter argues that China has been working incrementally but consistently
since the turn of the century to shape in its favour the evolution of the global
political-economic system, including the public health sector. How does the
West respond to this China challenge?

Chapter 4, titled 'China's Health Policy in Covid Times', takes stock of
what China has done so far to tackle the Covid-19 pandemic, at home and
abroad. It seeks answers to the following questions: What are the challenges
the country faces? What has China done to meet the challenge of a new health
order, an order in which it needs to strike a balance between championing
traditional Chinese medicine while using modern therapeutics? Above all,
how has the country emerged as one of the leading producers of medicinal
drugs and equipment? What makes the rise of China as the 'pharmacy of the
world'? What sort of policies has the country adopted to enhance its healthcare
provisions? In the process of reaching out to the outside world, how has the
country regulated its standards in order to harmonise with others, including
those standards in the field of traditional Chinese medicine? Last but not least,
how has the country's imposition of a zero-Covid policy for three years and its
sudden ditching affected the goodwill of the HSR?

Chapter 5, titled 'China's Vaccine Diplomacy and Health Governance',
looks critically at China's vaccine diplomacy, tracing its reach to Africa during
Covid times. This diplomacy contains an interesting new feature: the contributions made by the private sector and individuals. Since the 1960s, China
has been extending medical aid to African countries, including the dispatch
of medical teams. Covid-19 has provided China with a chance to consolidate
this tie. The country has exported large quantities of Covid vaccines and health

equipment to the continent and has helped to build many medical facilities in collaboration with the African Union. Apart from building transportation infrastructure like roads and railways, the provision of healthcare has become a prominent feature of China's development aid. In what ways has this new wave of development tested the efficacy of the HSR? How has this development shaped China's participation in global health governance, especially in its interactions with the World Health Organization? Can Africa produce enough vaccines to meet local needs in the near future, with the help of China, India, and countries in the West?

Chapter 6, titled 'Patient Rights vs Patent Rights', asks: What are patient rights? Are they human rights? What are patent rights? Are they monopolies in disguise? The debates between advocates of these two sets of rights are not new, but they have reached a new pitch as a result of the outbreak of Covid-19, leading to the scrambling for medicines by governments to save lives. The rise of China as a major power in global health affairs has added a new dimension to the debates. What are China's views on these debates? This chapter argues that China tilts towards favouring patient rights for developmental and ideological reasons. Its recognition of patient rights as human rights is in line with the views harboured by many developing countries and by international health bodies such as the WHO. This Chinese stance, however, is at odds with the views expressed by most, if not all, Western countries which hold the majority shares of the world's patent rights. How can the chasm between the two sets of rights be bridged? Can they coexist with each other in some way? How has China's HSR contributed to the easing or tightening of the tensions between the two opposing camps?

Chapter 7, titled 'Sino–US Rivalry: The Politics of Health', asks: Can China and the US work together to tackle global health problems? If so, what can they do? Bilateral relations between them have plummeted to new lows not seen since the days of Mao Zedong. Both countries have, however, recently identified global health as one of the areas in which they can cooperate for the benefit of both and for the world. Can collaboration in this area become a fresh start for building better relations, or will it be overwhelmed by a host of rivalries in the strategic, political, economic, and ideological fields. What and where is the key to turn enmity to amity? How do the two countries view each other? What are the structural problems besetting their relationship? How does the BRI, with its health component, stand between them? From China's point of view, it needs to take serious measures to protect itself from the relentless pressure exerted by the US. The country has adopted the so-called 'dual circulation' economic strategy to deal with this external pressure. What is this strategy? Will it work?

The concluding chapter, Chapter 8, brings together the findings of the previous chapters to explore the problems and prospects of the HSR. It argues that the HSR – an integral part of the modern Silk Road – has the potential to contribute substantially towards making a sustainable recovery and development for low-income countries, which have been suffering disproportionally from the scourge of Covid-19. Other factors that might slow down the world economy include the impact of China's adoption and sudden ditching of its zero-Covid policy and the war in Ukraine. China's return to the global supply chain after three years of isolation due to the pandemic, and the expansion of its BRI to the Global Development Initiative might help to redress the imbalance of wealth distribution between the rich and the poor in the world and to build global peace. Or would it? To what extent? As a conclusion, the chapter reviews the efficacy of geo-developmentalism as a theoretical tool to scrutinise the HSR.

NOTES

1. Gerald Chan, *Understanding China's new diplomacy: silk roads and bullet trains* (Cheltenham, UK, and Northampton, MA, USA: Edward Elgar Publishing, 2018).
2. Gerald Chan, *China's maritime Silk Road: advancing global development?* (Cheltenham, UK, and Northampton, MA, USA: Edward Elgar Publishing, 2020).
3. Gerald Chan, *China's digital Silk Roads: setting standards, powering growth* (Cheltenham, UK, and Northampton, MA, USA: Edward Elgar Publishing, 2022).
4. See: https:// www .scientificamerican .com/ article/ human -viruses -can -jump -into -animals -too -sowing -the -seeds -of -future -epidemics/ #: ~: text = In %20fact %2C %20since %20the %201980s ,including %20viruses %2C %20fungi %20and %20bacteria (accessed 13 February 2023).
5. It has been reported that in the written history of China, there have been some 1700 recorded incidents of great epidemics, roughly about once every two to three years on average. Jiang Yonghong, *Zhongguo yimiao bainian, 1919–2019* [*One hundred years of Chinese vaccines, 1919–2019*] (Hong Kong: Kaifang shudian, 2021), p. xiii.
6. See: https:// www .mfa .gov .cn/ ce/ cggb// eng/ xwdt/ t1375064 .htm (accessed 11 August 2022).
7. See: http://2017.beltandroadforum.org/english/n100/2017/0410/c22-45-3.html (accessed 23 February 2022).
8. See: https:// m .gmw .cn/ baijia/ 2021 -04/ 20/ 34776016 .html (accessed 2 June 2022).
9. Sourced mainly from Cao Jiahan, 'Toward a Health Silk Road: China's proposal for global health cooperation', *China Quarterly of International Strategic Studies*, Singapore, Vol. 6, No. 1 (2020), pp. 21–6.
10. See: https:// apps .who .int/ iris/ bitstream/ handle/ 10665/ 206614/ WPRO _2016 _DPM_003_eng.pdf?sequence=1&isAllowed=y (accessed 12 August 2022).
11. 'Development of China's public health as an essential element of human rights', White Paper, Information Office, State Council, PRC, September 2017.

12. See: https://www.mfa.gov.cn/ce/ceegy//eng/zgyw/t1756887.htm (accessed 30 May 2022).
13. See 'China Connects', International Institute for Strategic Studies, London, https://chinaconnects.iiss.org/ (accessed 15 May 2023).
14. 'BRI promotes inclusive globalization, peace', *China Daily*, Hong Kong ed., 1–2 July 2023, p. 4; 'China's Belt and Road Initiative to pursue "small but beautiful" projects as strategy turns 10', *South China Morning Post*, Hong Kong, 14 March 2023.
15. See: https://marketnews.com/mni-brief-china-will-look-to-belt-road-amid-trade-tensions (accessed 19 August 2023). For some details of 15 major projects, see *Zhongguo yidaiyilu nianjian* [*Yearbook of China's Belt and Road Initiative*] (Beijing: China Commerce and Trade Press, 2019) pp. 410–14.
16. See https://MarketNews.com.
17. 'BRI, as global public goods, fosters South–South cooperation', *China Daily*, Hong Kong ed., 1 August 2023, p. 18.
18. *China Daily*, August 2023.
19. 'China's Belt and Road Initiative to pursue "small but beautiful" projects as strategy turns 10'.
20. Shaun Lin, Naoko Shimazu, and James D. Sidaway, 'Theorising from the Belt and Road Initiative', *Asia Pacific Viewpoint*, Wellington, New Zealand, Vol. 62, No. 3 (December 2021), pp. 261–9.
21. In Jeremy Garlick, *The impact of China's Belt and Road Initiative: from Asia to Europe* (London: Routledge, 2019).
22. Garlick, 2019, Chapter 2.

2. Building Silk Roads: land, sea, digital, health

Confucius (551–479 BCE) states: there is a need to assign the correct name (*ye bi zhengming hu* 必也正名乎, the rectification of names); if the name is not assigned correctly, then one cannot speak smoothly and reasonably (*ming buzheng ze yan bushuen* 名不正则言不顺).[1] The leaders in Beijing probably rejoiced over picking 'the Silk Road' as the name for China's foreign policy. The name brings back great pride and fond memories of the past, for China and the countries and peoples who have been associated with it. Those were the days when China was a grand civilisation, rich and powerful, both materially and culturally. These days, the term 'modern Silk Roads' has come to be used by the Chinese authorities to rebrand, repackage, and relaunch the country's foreign relations.

This chapter sets the HSR against the backdrop of the BRI, which is primarily composed of the four Silk Roads: overland, maritime, digital, and health. The chapter brings these four components together to form a more complete picture of China's drive to develop, both domestically and globally. It argues that the *digital* component underpins the development of the other three. They work together holistically, however, to form a unique 'infrastructure of development', in contrast to the 'infrastructure of democracy' which has been developed over the past centuries by the West. As a component working at a critical juncture, the HSR affects in a major way the outcomes of the development of the other three. The Covid-19 pandemic is a case in point. The latter part of the chapter discusses the development of telehealth in China, including internet hospitals – a new venture at the forefront of medical innovation where technology meets healthcare.

To many students of oriental and medieval studies, the old Silk Roads call to mind images of the halcyon days of trade and cultural exchange among peoples and societies across Eurasia, maritime Asia, and the east coast of Africa. The Silk Road 'conjures up a hazy image of a caravan of camels laden with silk on a dusty desert track, reaching from China to Rome'.[2] It is not a single road, but multiple routes that crisscrossed Eurasia and provided 'a chain of markets that traded between east and west'.[3] The current leaders of China probably have serendipitously made effective use of this imagery to demonstrate China's soft powers to the outside world. The various major components of the modern Silk

Roads have neatly captured the important facets of many external relations. The overland, maritime, digital, and health Silk Roads are representative terms that signpost these major facets (Figure 2.1). Each of these can be teased out individually and analytically, and then assembled and reassembled in various ways to take the forms of trade, finance, physical connections and virtual links, people-to-people exchanges, and so on.

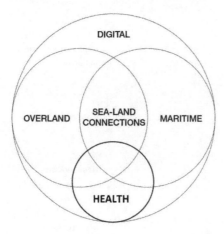

Figure 2.1   *The four major components of the new Silk Roads: land, sea, digital, health*

THE INFRASTRUCTURE OF DEVELOPMENT

The BRI is a diplomatic move that has helped showcase China's worldview. Its manifestation carries many past legacies. It has deep roots in the country's cross-border activities in the global political economy during the dynasties. Western perspectives and practices of the global political economy, on the other hand, started with European modernisation around the 1500s and have continued moving forward to the present day. They have formed a dominating force driving the economics and politics of the world, coinciding with European colonisation around the world through maritime conquests and land grabs, forging unequal trade relations, and sustaining post-imperialism in various ways. The two major sets of perspectives and practices – the East (China in this case) and the West – although divergent in many ways, are inevitably linked. Sometimes they work with each other and sometimes against, but most of the time they interact, bringing about a coexistence in which one contains and sustains the other, quite like the idea of yin and yang in Chinese philosophy. The coexistence is sometimes warm and sometimes frosty. Figure

2.2 shows a model of their connections and their different structures of development. In September 2021 President Xi Jinping proposed a new initiative called the Global Development Initiative, which has a strong connection with the BRI. We shall discuss its prospects in greater detail in the concluding chapter.

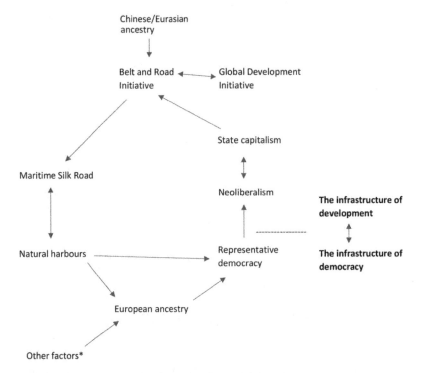

Note: *Including economics, institutions, and culture. Natural harbours are a geographic construct.
Source: The lower half of this figure depicting the 'infrastructure of democracy' is sourced from John Gerring et al., *The deep roots of modern democracy* (Cambridge: Cambridge University Press, 2022), p. 6. The upper half on the 'infrastructure of development' is my own construction.

Figure 2.2   The deep structure of the global political economy

China's HSR grows largely out of the country's health diplomacy, which has received relatively little attention from China watchers when compared to the country's political and economic diplomacy, for several reasons. First, China's health diplomacy is low-key. The amount of its health aid is small, and the issue does not seem to be high on the agenda in comparison with other kinds of Chinese aid and investment, such as the huge tickets for infrastructure. Second, the country has had relatively little advanced health technology to share with other countries until very recently. It has just begun to apply hi-tech knowledge such as telemedicine and mobile healthcare on a large scale to support and promote its healthcare system. Traditional Chinese medicine has, however, been practised in the country over several millennia, but it is an Indigenous medical discipline that is vastly different from modern Western medicine. Although widely used in Chinese societies, especially on the China mainland and in overseas Chinese communities, Chinese medicine as a discipline has not yet made any significant breakthroughs globally as a body of medical knowledge and as a medical practice. It has now acquired some increasing, yet limited, recognition in other parts of the world beyond the Chinese diaspora. (See Chapter 4 for more on Chinese medicine.) Third, China's health diplomacy has had relatively little impact on the political and economic interests of the West, again until very recently, when China expanded the reach of its BRI, bringing some aspects of health assistance to various parts of the world. Traditionally, China's foreign health assistance has been targeted at some poor countries in the Global South, particularly Africa, for political and ideological reasons, and it still does (to be further discussed in Chapter 5).

The use of the term 'Health Silk Road' makes nostalgic connections with other components of China's BRI. It has acquired a geopolitical and geo-economic flavour beyond health issues. HSR now carries a new meaning, especially when it is viewed in the context of China's continuing economic rise, the rapid spread of Covid-19, the emergence of virus variants since 2020, and other possible outbreaks of disease in the future. The health component is increasingly linked to the digital component through the rapid advancements made in healthcare delivery using digital means, such as the popular use of telemedicine or telehealth. The outreach of the HSR has shown its increasing linkages with the other three components of the BRI, particularly with the digital Silk Road in a fast-evolving digital world.

The delivery of physical commodities such as medical equipment and drugs and the movement of medical personnel still require physical transportation, so the efficient operation of the overland and maritime Silk Roads (in terms of the use of container trucks and freight trains, and shipping and air transportation) is essential to the working of at least the physical delivery aspect of the HSR. The speedy distribution of huge volumes of Chinese vaccines and medical supplies and equipment around the world in 2020 to combat Covid-19 is a case in point. China's transportation and logistics infrastructure and its thriving e-commerce activities have played a significant part in facilitating this export and distribution (more in Chapter 5). Figure 2.1 shows the linkages among the four major components of the BRI. One of the manifestations of these linkages is telehealth, a product of the integration of healthcare provisions with digital technology.

TELEHEALTH: WHEN TECHNOLOGY MEETS HEALTHCARE

Telehealth – the use of technology to meet health needs remotely – is not entirely new. It has been practised in some countries for decades.[4] But Covid-19 greatly accelerated its use in a more dramatic fashion and in a transformative way both in terms of the scope, scale, and speed of delivery and in terms of the development of new drugs and medical devices. Digital technology has changed the way we live and work. In numerous ways, telehealth (known also as telemedicine, digital health or e-health) has changed substantially the relationship between patients, healthcare providers, and the healthcare system itself. During the Covid pandemic, telemedicine helped a great deal to preserve the use of personal protective equipment when they were in short supply, to minimise the chances of healthcare providers being infected, and to allow the monitoring of patients' conditions without putting them at risk by requiring their attendance at traditional medical settings.

The WHO has defined telehealth as 'delivery of health care services, where patients and providers are separated by distance. Telehealth uses information communication technology for the exchange of information for the diagnosis and treatment of diseases and injuries, research and evaluation, and for the continuing education of health professionals'.[5] The New Zealand Telehealth Forum has defined telehealth as 'health care delivered using digital technology where participants may be separated by time and/or distance'.[6] A group of Chinese medical researchers have said that 'telemedicine refers to the remote delivery of health care services with the use of modern communication technology'.[7] In China's case, these services include internet hospitals, online sales of drugs, artificial intelligence (AI)-based medical devices, big data, and medical robots, among other inventions and innovations. The two terms – telemedicine and telehealth – are often used interchangeably, although some medical professionals would like to make a distinction between them, referring telemedicine to clinical services while telehealth to a wider field that includes non-clinical services such as medical training, administrative meetings, and further medical education.[8]

For quite some time, the US has been working at the forefront of this field. One of the earliest uses of hospital-based telemedicine took place in the late 1950s and early 1960s in Nebraska, where a closed-circuit television was linked up with medical facilities.[9] Shortly before the outbreak of Covid-19 in late 2019, the use of telehealth in American hospitals had grown from 35 per cent (of hospitals fully or partially implementing telehealth systems) in 2010 to 76 per cent in 2017.[10] McKinsey & Company, a business consultancy, pointed out that the consumer adoption of telehealth in the US during Covid times had skyrocketed from 11 per cent of consumers in 2019 to 46 per cent in July 2021. Many American hospitals had used telehealth to replace cancelled healthcare visits.[11]

Covid-19 has also changed the face of the European response to healthcare. In March 2021 the European Commission initiated a programme costing €5.1 billion for digital transformation of the EU health sector and to prepare for future cross-border pandemic outbreaks.[12] The Commission's Communication on Digital Transformation of Health and Care has worked consistently to gain the support and momentum in empowering citizens and to build a healthier society through the greater use of digital technology. As a result, telehealth has established a strong foothold on the continent.

In Asia, a number of countries have been pioneers in introducing telehealth. They include, among others,[13] China, Japan, South Korea, Indonesia, India, Singapore, Malaysia, and the Philippines. China has been spearheading the move. The telehealth industry in China has grown by leaps and bounds, fuelled by its rapid development of information and communication technologies (ICT), especially in tech applications. Statista, a data-research provider, estimates that the market size of the telehealth industry in China was 41 million yuan in 2015, rising year on year to 130 million yuan in 2019.[14] This happened before the outbreak of Covid-19. During the rapid spread of the virus from 2020 to 2022, the market size exploded, and it is estimated to reach $50 billion by 2025,[15] against the US's market size of $35 billion in the same year.[16] China will have surpassed the US as the leading telehealth market by the end of 2023. In terms of the overall healthcare industry (including telehealth), the market size was 1.93 trillion yuan in 2010, rising swiftly over the years to reach 7.82 trillion yuan (US$1.1 trillion) in 2019.[17] An investment firm in Singapore estimates that the entire healthcare industry in China will reach over 10 trillion yuan by 2024 and over 17 trillion yuan by 2030.[18]

Several factors may have contributed to the growth of e-health in China. These include socio-economic factors and institutional supports. The socio-economic factors include such things as an ageing population, a rising per-capita disposable income, an increasing prevalence of chronic diseases such as stroke, heart disease, and cancer, and a growing awareness of the importance of hygiene among the general public.[19] The outbreak of Covid-19 has magnified the impact of these factors. From an institutional perspective, many private information technology (IT) companies have started to provide the necessary tech supports and financial platforms, and the central and regional governments have prepared the necessary legal framework and offered financial incentives. Together, all these aspects seem to have worked well to facilitate a speedy development.

As in many other areas of modernisation, China started late in developing telehealth. The reform and opening up of the country beginning in the 1980s

Table 2.1   China's digital health policies since 2014

Date	Policy	Issuing office	Objectives
2014 August	Opinions	National Health and Family Planning Commission	To promote the use of telemedicine
2015 January	Technical guidelines for the establishment of a telemedicine information system	National Health and Family Planning Commission	To build a uniform national telemedicine service network
2016 October	'Healthy China 2030'	State Council	To boost support to the health-tech industry
2018 April	'Internet Plus Medicine & Health'	State Council	To build an architecture for integrating IT and healthcare
2019 August	Project launch	National Healthcare Security Administration	To launch an e-medical insurance scheme
2019 October	Guidance	National Healthcare Security Administration	To promote 'Internet+'*
2020 May	Statement	National Health Commission**	To direct provincial governments to set regulations on managing e-healthcare
2022 April	Information regulation in the 14th Five-Year Plan	Cyberspace Administration of China	To connect and balance regional developments, using IT to promote e-health management

Notes: * The 'Internet+' is a five-year health plan to integrate cloud computing, big data, and the Internet of Things with a variety of industries.
** Replacing the National Health and Family Planning Commission, under the State Council.
Source: Adapted from https://www.china-briefing.com/news/understanding-chinas-interne t-healthcare-and-opportunities-for-foreign-investors/ (accessed 24 August 2022) and other internet sources.

has generated a congenial environment for nurturing innovation and rewarding those who show initiative, with the accompanying risks and opportunities. It was after China's entry into the World Trade Organization (WTO) in 2001 that the country began to pay increasing attention to the development of digital health. Table 2.1 highlights some of the major policies that the government has adopted to guide this development.

Chinese IT entrepreneurs are ambitious and aggressive. They are eager to exploit the opportunities made available by a relatively relaxed political and business environment to explore, start up, and expand their businesses not only in e-commerce, communications, and entertainment, but also in financial

Table 2.2   *Three main private digital healthcare providers in China, 2021*

	JD Health	AliHealth	Ping An Good Doctor
Year founded	2017	2004	2014
Market capital (Hong Kong, billions of US dollars, September 2021)	240	170	63
Online retail pharmacy	Yes (90% of revenue)	Yes (98% of revenue)	Yes (54% of revenue)
Online consultation	Yes	Yes	Yes
Insurance	'Family Doctor Insurance'	Piloting direct insurance billing (with AliPay)	Commercial insurance coverage (incl. 1k+ corporations)
Comparative strength	No. of pharmacies	No. of users	No. of hospitals

Sources: Adapted from https://www.youtube.com/watch?v=NMRXCKIE9Ck (accessed 24 August 2022) and other internet sources.

services and now healthcare facilities. They make good use of the latest IT applications designed for the purpose. Alibaba, Tencent, Baidu, Xiaomi, and JD.com are a few highly successful examples. Many Chinese digital health and wellness companies started to appear in the early 2010s. According to Omdia, a research company based in London, in 2020 Chinese startups attracted US$1.4 billion of financing, compared to US$2.4 billion generated by their US counterparts. Together, the two countries account for 90 per cent of global investment in medical AI startups.[20] As of June 2022, there were 1758 health-tech startups in China.[21] Some of them focus on internet hospital services. Examples of internet hospital unicorns (those with valuations of a billion dollars or above) in 2019 include We Doctor Group, Haodf.com, Chunyuyisheng.com, Miaoshou.com, Medlinker, Hellan Health, and www.dxy.cn.[22] Table 2.2 compares three leading private e-health providers in the country.

At present, 89 per cent of healthcare professionals in the country use tele-health and 73 per cent of them administer telemedicine.[23] The country has 4.29 million licensed doctors as of 2021,[24] serving an ageing population of 1.4 billion people. Medical consultations provided through Haodf.com, one of China's largest internet health platforms, increased by 75 per cent between January and March 2020.[25] New investments in China's internet health market stood at 37.9 billion yuan (US$5.7 billion) in 2019, up from 4.5 billion yuan (US$675 million) in 2013.[26]

Other Asian countries are playing catch-up in setting up digital healthcare platforms. These include Mecin of Japan,[27] Standigm of South Korea,[28]

DocOnline of India, Haldoc and Good Doctor of Indonesia, Noah of Singapore, Speedoc of Malaysia, KonsultaMD of the Philippines, and Doctor Raksa of Thailand, among many others. Those in Japan and South Korea are more advanced in their development than the others.

African countries have recently started to develop telehealth. South Africa, Nigeria,[29] and Egypt are leading the way. The first continental-wide conference on telehealth was held online in mid-2021, and the second Africa telehealth conference was held in Cairo at the end of 2022.[30] In Latin America, Covid-19 has also stimulated interest in exploring telehealth services, with Brazil and Argentina leading the way.[31] In the Middle East, telehealth and telemedicine platforms are gaining popularity in Saudi Arabia and the United Arab Emirates.[32]

CHINA'S INTERNET HOSPITALS[33]

The development of internet hospitals in China gives a good picture of the overall development of telehealth and telemedicine in the country. Like the situation in many countries, there are two types of internet hospitals in China[34]: (1) the 'hospital + internet' type: these are physical healthcare institutions that provide internet hospital services; and (2) the 'internet + hospital' type: independent internet hospitals whose medical services rely on physical medical entities, including hospitals jointly established with digital companies. The major difference between the two is the different emphasis on hospitals or the internet as the basis of the services that they provide.

The first internet hospital in China was set up in 2014 in the southern province of Guangdong.[35] In December 2015, Guizhou, a province in the south-west, issued the first implementation plan for a pilot scheme on internet hospitals. The ensuing years saw some ups and downs in the number of startups of internet hospitals due to murky government regulations and to user doubts about the reliability of such services. The publication of an access policy for internet hospitals issued by the central government in 2018, followed by documents setting out implementation rules, spurred a resurgence of these hospitals. In 2019 there were 197 internet hospitals, a huge jump from 26 a year earlier. The number reached 1004 at the end of 2020,[36] 1600 in August 2021,[37] and over 1900 at the end of 2021.[38] According to Xinhua news agency, nearly 49 million people took online diagnosis and treatments in 2020.[39] Covid-19 has created a heavy demand for telemedicine services in the country. The internet hospitals provide guidance to patients seeking appropriate medical treatment and meet the urgent needs of chronically ill patients through online medical check-ups, payment, and drug dispensation.

At present, there are three major telehealth networks in the country: the Golden Health Network, the International MedioNet of China, and the

People's Liberation Army telemedicine network. According to a market insider,[40] the research and application in the field are still at an early stage, but there are heavy demands fuelled by a huge, ageing population and the rapid development of IT, especially 5G communication. The industry has a lot of room for further expansion and improvements. The same is true for many similar markets in other parts of the world.

As countries develop telehealth mostly on their own, the WHO is concerned about the proliferation of different medical and ethical standards and about the issue of equity in accessing telehealth services from different sectors of society, especially marginalised communities (the physically and mentally impaired, for example) in a digitally divided world. To address these concerns, the WHO has teamed up with the International Telecommunication Union to develop a global standard and has recently published a joint report on the issue.[41] The standard developed provides a list of technical requirements intended for adoption by member states of the WHO as regulations or legislation. The world body encourages healthcare professionals and manufacturers to implement the requirements voluntarily.[42]

China is now leading the way in adopting digital health technology, according to a survey of healthcare professionals in 15 countries around the world – the 2019 Future Health Index from Philips, a Dutch multinational. The Index also shows that emerging countries are more enthusiastic than other countries in deploying AI to support their healthcare system.[43] China started late in this journey but has moved faster and further than the West in setting up a unified digital health ecosystem, leapfrogging many early stages of development. This situation bears some similarities to the skipping of the use of PCs in communication by jumping straight to the use of mobile phones, and to the skipping of the use of credit cards to the use of digital currency.[44] It has happened in China, and it is happening in many African countries.[45]

CONCLUSION

As an important component of the BRI, the HSR aims to connect countries by building a health infrastructure to generate mutual benefits for China and the host countries concerned. A critical test of this development is what China has done and the extent to which it will share its knowledge of healthcare and its experience in the field with others, especially with developing countries. Future development depends on, among other things, what and how countries in the Global South will receive from China in return for reciprocal offers. It will also depend on how other donor countries in the West react to China's health assistance. What will China do to transfer its technology in telehealth? We shall return to discuss this area of research and development, as well as capacity building, in Chapter 5 when we focus on vaccine diplomacy. In the meantime, let us turn our attention to the global structure of public health, where the HSR is seeded, in the next chapter.

NOTES

1. See: https://www.lhp.sdu.edu.cn/__local/1/ED/A4/40BC1CC E8C0878E5E F0AA83622F_E5978975_15E99F.pdf (accessed 2 March 2023). Partly my translation.
2. Valerie Hansen, *The Silk Road: a new history* (Oxford: Oxford University Press, 2012), jacket.
3. Hansen, 2012.
4. 'WHO–ITU global standard for accessibility of telehealth service', WHO and ITU, 2022, p. vii.
5. WHO and ITU, 2022.
6. See: https://www.telehealth.org.nz/health-provider/what-is-telehealth/ (accessed 12 February 2022).
7. See: https://www.ncbi.nlm.nih.gov/pmc/articles/PMC7647817/ (accessed 13 February 2022).
8. See: https://chironhealth.com/blog/telemedicine-vs-telehealth-whats-the-difference/ (accessed 16 August 2022).
9. See: https://www.ncbi.nlm.nih.gov/books/NBK207141/#:~:text=Probably %20one %20of %20the %20earliest ,State %20Hospital %20for %20psychiatric %20consultations (accessed 24 August 2022).
10. See: https://www.aha.org/factsheet/telehealth (accessed 15 August 2022).
11. See: https://www.mckinsey.com/industries/healthcare-systems-and-services/our -insights/telehealth-a-quarter-trillion-dollar-post-covid-19-reality (accessed 15 August 2022).
12. See: https://www.healthcareitnews.com/news/emea/european-digital-health -revolution-wake-covid-19 (accessed 10 June 2023).
13. For a study of the development of telehealth in Japan and South Korea, see: https://healthadvancesblog.com/2022/05/04/digital-health-in-japan-and-korea -where-is-it-heading/ (accessed 27 August 2022).
14. See: https://www.statista.com/statistics/1245525/china-telemedicine-market -size/ (accessed 24 August 2022).
15. See: https://www.cnbc.com/how-china-turned-to-telehealth-during-the-coronavirus/ (accessed 24 August 2022).
16. See CNBC.com, 'How China turned'.
17. See: https://www.china-briefing.com/news/china-investment-outlook-telemedicine -digital-healthcare-industry/ (accessed 16 August 2022).
18. See MoneyWiseSmart, 2 October 2021, https://www.youtube.com/watch?v= NMRXCKIE9Ck (accessed 24 August 2022).
19. See MoneyWiseSmart, 2 October 2021.
20. As reported by the *Financial Times*, https://www.ft.com/content/c1fe6fbf-8a87 -4328-9e75-816009a07a59 (accessed 30 January 2023).
21. HealthTech Startups in China, Tracxn (accessed 25 August 2022).
22. 'Internet hospitals in China: the new step into digital healthcare', Deloitte, 2021, p. 13.
23. See: https://www.kcl.ac.uk/news/chinas-digital-mental-health-services-outpacing -regulation (accessed 25 August 2022).

24. See: https://www.statista.com/statistics/279326/number-of-licensed-doctors-in-china/ (accessed 30 January 2023).
25. Fastdata极数 (ifastdata.com) (accessed 27 August 2022).
26. See Fastdata.
27. See: https://micin.jp/en (accessed 27 August 2022).
28. See: https://tracxn.com/explore/HealthTech-Startups-in-South-Korea (accessed 27 August 2022).
29. See: https://www.afdb.org/en/news-and-events/africa-investment-forum-attracts-us-trade-and-development-agency-support-nigerian-telehealth-provider-55885 (accessed 2 May 2023).
30. See: https://www.africa-telehealth.com/ (accessed 2 May 2023).
31. See: https://www.medigraphic.com/cgi-bin/new/resumenI.cgi?IDARTICULO=93574 (accessed 2 May 2023).
32. See: https://www.grandviewresearch.com/industry-analysis/middle-east-africa-telehealth-market-report#:~:text=In%20countries%20such%20as%20Saudi,increase%20in%20cyber%20security%20issues (accessed 20 August 2023).
33. This section draws heavily from Li Yushan et al., 'COVID-19 and internet hospital development in China', 2 June 2022, https://www.mdpi.com/2673-3986/3/2/21/htm (accessed 16 August 2022).
34. 'Internet hospitals in China', p. 8.
35. See: http://www.chinadaily.com.cn/world/2015-07/23/content_21396510.htm (accessed 16 August 2022).
36. Li, 'COVID-19 and internet hospital development in China'.
37. 'Over 1600 internet hospitals established in China', *Xinhua*, 20 August 2021.
38. Chambers and Partners, 'Digital Healthcare 2022, China, Global practice guides', https://practiceguides.chambers.com/practice-guides/digital-healthcare-2022/china/trends-and-developments/O11012 (accessed 25 August 2022).
39. 'Over 1600 internet hospitals established in China'.
40. See: http://www.frostchina.com/?p=3809 (accessed 16 August 2022).
41. WHO and ITU, 2022.
42. See: https://www.who.int/publications/i/item/9789240050464 (accessed 28 March 2023).
43. Philips, 'Transforming healthcare experiences – Future Health Index report 2019', https://www.philips.com/a-w/about/news/future-health-index/reports/2019/transforming-healthcare-experiences.html (accessed 25 August 2022).
44. See Gerald Chan, *China's digital Silk Road: setting standards, powering growth* (Cheltenham, UK, and Northampton, MA, USA, 2022), pp. 66–90.
45. Chan, 2022, pp. 98–99.

3. The global structure of public health

Global public health refers to public health issues that have come to the fore in the global environment,[1] such as the emergence of infectious diseases and their impact, control, and prevention. Global public health has its particular focus and interests but it does not exist in a vacuum. It works within a greater universe – the global political economy. It is heavily conditioned by the power structure of this greater universe, especially when viewed from the perspective of structural realism in the study of International Relations, apart from its value systems and its modes of reasoning.[2] So, what is this global political economy? In simple terms, it is the sum total of the interactions between politics and economics at the global level. It involves important actors such as the state, the market, and multinationals, among others, as well as the interactions among these actors at many levels, from the individual to the global. It is therefore highly complex, considering the many units involved in interacting with each other in numerous ways at multiple levels in the system. To unpack this complexity, one needs to look deeply into the structure of the global system in which the global political economy is embedded. This would then permit a better understanding of how things work, including the global health system and China's HSR.

One way to do this is to examine how power is exercised within the system and what consequences ensue. To carry out this examination, I propose to start by looking at some major concepts that underlie the growth of our knowledge and understanding of the basic constituencies of the global system – capitalism, imperialism, and neoliberalism. Here, our analysis relies mainly on a reading of the literature prevalent in the West. This is because the Western tradition has played a pivotal role in shaping the development of modern international relations, more so than any other traditions, such as the Chinese, Hindu, Islamic, or Persian civilisations. It does not mean, however, that these other traditions and civilisations have little to contribute in reaching a more complete understanding of the global political economy. They are indeed important agents and drivers in international relations in their own right. The rise of China in contemporary times, for example, has posed a huge challenge to the existing international system, which has been dominated, controlled, and maintained by the West since the Industrial Revolution and Enlightenment. One of the great challenges facing this global (read Western) order in recent times is the BRI, China's flagship foreign policy, which can be seen as a primary case of 'globalisation with Chinese characteristics'.[3] There are also other reasons for relying on Western literature, such as the availability of sources and the preferences of readers.

This chapter lays out the global political economy as a context in which to examine China's participation in the global health system. First, what is global public health? What are its origins and development? What features characterise its structure? To understand the structure of global public health and its evolution, we need to cast a wider scope of investigation to comprehend the bigger picture of which the structure of global public health forms a part. This chapter chooses to focus on the three major components of the global political economy: capitalism, imperialism, and neoliberalism. Together, they effectively capture the essence of the relationships between and among states and other major non-state actors in international relations. What is the nature, substance, and linkages of these components? How have they evolved over time? Is the current global public health structure under stress because of the erosion of its foundation? If so, in what way? Are there modifications, substitutes, or alternatives to this deep structure? If so, what are they and what is their purpose? These questions are not entirely new; but attempting to understand their evolving nature could help anchor the analysis carried out in this book.

The development of Western political thought has embraced, among other things, a common theme – the issue of (in)equality, with a largely hidden assumption that there is a (universal) standard of civilisation enshrined in Western values. It is, from an opposing point of view, racism and discrimination in disguise. Or is it? Is fair trade and the spread of the (Western) standard of civilisation that common theme, a thesis so eloquently espoused and depicted by the English School of International Relations?[4] Is the West, led by the US, now receding to the adoption of trade protectionism and neonationalism to counter the rise of emerging economies, China in particular, thereby triggering a shift in the balance of power, economics, and ideologies?[5]

THE STRUCTURE OF CAPITALISM

Capitalism in the modern era emerged from the collapse of feudalism in the 16th century as a new way of organising society and its economy. The development of industrialisation and the accompanying growth of private ownership (from land- and asset-based to labour-based) gave rise to the beginning of capitalism. Capitalism has become an economic system based on the private ownership of the means of production and of their operation for profit.[6] It leads to the accumulation of wealth in the hands of the capitalists. It defines what constitutes 'fair' play and 'fair' pay. In simple terms, capitalist systems are controlled by market forces where capital goods are owned by businesses and individuals.[7] In a traditional capitalist economy, assets such as factories, mines, and railroads are typically owned and controlled by private hands. In contemporary times, asset management – the practice of increasing total wealth over time by acquiring, maintaining, and trading investments that have the potential to grow in value[8] – has become the holy grail of capitalism, in what political economist Brett Christophers has called rentier capitalism.[9] Labour, on the other hand, can be purchased through wages,[10] a major advancement over the ownership of slaves.

Today, capitalism serves as an economic system that relies on a (relatively) free market to determine the most efficient way to allocate resources and set prices based on supply and demand, with minimal government intervention. It has evolved into neoliberalism. Socialism, generally regarded as the opposing system, is one where there is little or no free market, and where the allocation of resources is determined by a central authority.[11] Understood in this way, capitalism and socialism occupy positions at the opposite ends of a continuum. In between both ends and along the continuum, there exist various forms of hybrid systems with a different mix of capitalist and socialist ways of doing things. From this perspective, China has been moving progressively along this continuum from socialism to capitalism, with varying degrees of adjustments over time, in a fluid hybrid form, especially since its adoption of the reform and opening up in the 1980s.

China's current economic system has been labelled as socialism with Chinese characteristics (by Chinese officials) or state capitalism (by many outside observers). There are also other labels, such as autocratic capitalism, developmental capitalism, and so on. In the main, the party-state is in effective control, while allowing increasing space for private enterprises to function and thrive. According to some free-market thinkers, however, the scope and speed of change from public to private are limited.

THE STRUCTURE OF IMPERIALISM

How has the world of capitalism been spreading, especially to new territories where unequal development is seen to have been established? The theory of imperialism, among others, effectively helps explain the cause and consequences of such unequal development. Imperialism refers to the overwhelming dominance of some states over others. This asymmetric relationship in power – political, economic, and social – generates and sustains a system of exploitation. Imperialism is exercised through a forced acquisition of assets and territories – in both physical and social space – through the exercise of a combination of military, political, economic, and religious powers in colonial expansion. It has been used as a theory, a doctrine, a strategy, a practice, a policy, or an advocacy, legalised and legitimised by the norms and rules set up by the dominating states, first extraterritorially and then regionally and universally – sometimes successfully, sometimes not.[12]

The 'Doctrine of Discovery' has been used by competing colonial powers in Europe, in one way or another, as a 'legitimate' way to claim sovereign rights over non-Christian, native land in Africa and the Americas.[13] This doctrine can be traced back to the papal edict of the 15th century. It was only repudiated formally by the Vatican in March 2023 in response to calls made by Indigenous leaders of Canada during Pope Francis's visit a year earlier. Colonialism has a very long tail. The doctrine was still cited in the US Supreme Court as late as 2015,[14] and it extends beyond land. Some of the effects of discrimination and forced assimilation policies are still in place today.

Johan Galtung, a well-known Norwegian peace researcher, has eloquently depicted the structure of imperialism in modern times by using a simple model of a world consisting of two parts: the Core and the Periphery (or the developed and developing countries).[15] The Core can be visualised as consisting again of two parts: its own core and periphery. So is the Periphery which can be seen to be divided into its own core and periphery. Exploitation of the Periphery by the Core is exercised through a link (of harmony of interest) between the core of the Core and the core of the Periphery, so that resources from the periphery of the Periphery are being sucked and channelled through this link (based on unequal trading terms) to the core of the Core. This unequal exchange is sustained by the extraction of natural resources and the buying of primary produce at a cheap price from the Periphery while selling to it high-valued manufactured products and providing high-valued services from the Core. The core of the Periphery is sometimes labelled as the *comprador* class, which serves as a link or bridgehead between the Periphery and the Core. This class also serves useful functions as agents of modernisation and urbanisation for the Periphery,[16] while generating wealth for themselves and a few others in the process.

The outcome of this Core–Periphery relationship is that resources are being sucked from the periphery of the Periphery to the core of the Periphery and then, via the link (or bridgehead), to the core of the Core. And through the social welfare system within the Core (a system which is more advanced than a similar system in the Periphery), some of the resources accumulated in the core of the Core are being distributed or trickled down to the periphery of the Core. The Core can do this because of its dominating power, not only in politics and economics, but also in socialisation, education, science and technology, and other societal dimensions. As a result, the rich (Core) get richer and the poor (Periphery) get poorer. In other words, the wealth gap between the Global North and the Global South widens. According to the World Bank,[17] the poorest half of the world population has been getting only 2.3 per cent of the overall global wealth growth since 1995. The top 1 per cent of the world's population has been benefiting from high growth rates of 3 per cent to 9 per cent per year. This super-rich group captured 38 per cent of the total wealth increases between 1995 and 2021.

Apart from the link between the core of the Core and the core of the Periphery (in the simplified two-part world), this structure of imperialism is also sustained by the link(s) among the Core countries. These links are sustained by the so-called coalitions of allies in strategic terms and, to a lesser extent, close working relationships with partners. These coalitions, often led by the most powerful state of them all, then set the rules for the world, often called 'international law', to be adhered to by all other states. The English School of International Relations also refers to these rules and laws as the 'standard of civilisation'.[18] They are set by the major powers to be followed by all. However, the fruits of the international society, which are so created and reaped, may not be shared with developing countries or shared with them in a 'fair' way. These countries are regarded by the rich and powerful countries, formally or informally, openly or discreetly, as not belonging to 'the civilisation' club, and so they can be treated differently. For example, in a system of extraterritoriality, the colonial or imperial class can enjoy special privileges and legal protection denied to the locals. Within the area of extraterritoriality, legal jurisdiction lay in the hands of consular courts set up by the colonisers.[19] Fast-forward to the present, the use of domestic legislation by a power to sanction other countries is a modern application of this traditional practice, chastised by countries at the receiving end of these punishing sanctions.

An interesting point about this structure of imperialism is that, while the Core countries are in some coalition or partnership with each other, the vast majority of Periphery countries are not. Many of them are separated from each other, individually or in small groups. This configuration is known as the divide-and-rule principle, and it sustains the international division of labour that benefits largely the Core (rich) countries rather than the Periphery (poor) countries.

The trillion-dollar question for developing countries is: How to break this global chain of unequal exchange, this aggressive and exploitative relationship? There is no easy answer, to be sure. In the contemporary world, an international tax of one kind or another has been proposed to promote equity but hard to be formulated.[20] International aid has been put into practice, with some notable successes in helping the poor, but it has not been able to resolve the issue of worldwide poverty. On the contrary, the global wealth gap has been increasing. Galtung has suggested that developing countries (in the Periphery) should turn to self-reliance and self-help – to decouple from the Core and hence break that exploitative relationship. Another way is to adopt an import-substitution policy. To address the issue of the lack of connectivity between and among developing countries and to counter the divide-and-rule system, a complementary method is to develop such links. In other words, develop Periphery–Periphery or South–South cooperation.

China is still regarded as a developing country by the World Bank and other international organisations,[21] due to its relatively low average gross domestic product (GDP) per capita, its uneven development and distribution of wealth in different parts of the country, and the existence of pockets of abject poverty in some remote areas, especially in the west. A rising China can play a major role in promoting South–South cooperation. It can help raise the economic standards of many low-income countries through its BRI and HSR, and also through the Global Development Initiative (GDI), proposed in 2021. (We will discuss the GDI in the concluding chapter.)

Potentially, other large developing countries can help as well. Consider the BRICS (Brazil, Russia, India, China, and South Africa) emerging economies. Apart from China, Russia is now in a no-go position because of its focus on the war in Ukraine (as of 2023). Brazil has just turned the corner from an ultra-right government under Jair Bolsonaro to a socialist-leaning one under Luiz Inácio Lula da Silva. It needs time to rebuild. South Africa, the weakest link in the BRICS, is in domestic turmoil brought about by political corruption and power outages. India stands out as another possible strong country in a position to offer South–South help. The country, however, can only do so much given its own domestic priorities, in comparison with China's Belt and Road. India's rivalry with China means that it is more focused on building its sphere of influence in South Asia – its own backyard – in large part to counter China's increasing presence and influence in the region. India's behaviour is difficult to assess. It has a mind of its own, according to some India watchers. It sides with the Periphery, but has also maintained strategic relationships with Core countries in, for example, the Quad (consisting of the US, Australia, Japan, and India). At the same time, it tries hard to maintain its independent, non-aligned policy, a legacy of the past. This includes its independence from Great Britain and an inheritance of the Bandung Spirit of 1955, when non-aligned countries in the developing world tried to carve out a strategic space in international politics to protect and promote their national interests, called the New International Economic Order (NIEO) within the UN family. The NIEO has not been working well as a group, partly because of its huge size of almost 100 developing countries, partly because of a lack of coordination, and partly because of the absence of a strong leader. Seventy years after the formation of the NIEO born out of the Bandung Non-Aligned Movement and ten years after the launch of the BRI, China has now (as of 2023) become the second-largest economy in the world and the largest trader. Can China answer the leadership call so desperately needed to rally the developing world?

To compete with China in building infrastructure in the Global South and to increase their influence, the Core countries are now turning their attention to these nations to build better infrastructure. This time, they (the G7 wealthy countries, together with some emerging economies in the G20) return to Africa and the South Pacific, as partners rather than as big brothers. So China has potentially more competitors in the global infrastructure game.

In watching the rise of China, a question is often asked: When China becomes strong, will it behave like other rising powers and become imperialist? Chinese officials have repeatedly and consistently stressed that China will never become a hegemon. To some, however, China has become more aggressive in strategic areas such as the Taiwan Strait, the South China Sea, and the East China Sea. To others, China as a rising power has more interests to protect and promote, not unlike any other country in a similar situation. To them, China is more assertive rather than aggressive. Who is right, who is wrong? We have to wait and see. One thing about China is different: rising powers in modern times have all been Western powers. China is not. Will it therefore become an exception to the rule – that is, when China becomes strong, will it not become a hegemon?

THE STRUCTURE OF NEOLIBERALISM

Neoliberalism built on the shoulders of capitalism and imperialism to evolve into a political-economic philosophy in the latter days of the Cold War. It has been characterised by the economic policies of US President Ronald Reagan and British Prime Minister Margaret Thatcher. The driving force has been the military-industrial complex of the US working in tandem with Wall Street financiers to generate what has become known as the Washington consensus. At the heart of this consensus is free trade and the primacy of the market. Neoliberalists argue that such driving forces best serve to grow the economy. State intervention, to them, would be antithetic to growth.

Neoliberalism embraces pro-market policies in many forms and shapes in contemporary times. They include the elimination of price controls, the deregulation of capital markets, the lowering of trade barriers, and the reduction of state influence in the economy. Such a system is augmented through privatisation and austerity measures.[22]

Neoliberalists believe (in good faith or pretentiously, rightly or wrongly) that greater economic freedom leads to greater economic growth for society and greater social progress for individuals. Based on this assumption, they support free enterprise, competition, deregulation, and individual responsibility. They oppose the expansion of government intervention, increasing social welfare, and rising inflation.[23] As a product borne out of capitalism and imperialism, neoliberalism shares in large part the legacies, heritage, and logics of its predecessors. It has been deployed as a policy and a practice and promoted as a theory and an ideology. Its impact has been phenomenal, influencing many parts of the world, if not all.

Apparently, neoliberalism plays well for the rich and powerful, the industrialised and developed, but not for the developing world struggling to modernise and catch up. Does the idea of freedom so cherished by neoliberalism include the freedom to 'exploit' behind the façade of free trade and the opening up of overseas markets? Does it include the freedom not to be 'exploited'? The main sticking point is still the unequal terms of trade that sustain global inequality, in economics as well as in healthcare. From the perspective of the developing world, the system of patent rights that protects the interests of pharmaceutical companies can be viewed as a freeway leading to unequal terms of exchange through trade in medicinal products. The conflicts and debates over patent rights versus the right of patients to access affordable life-saving drugs have come to the fore of international concern during the Covid-19 pandemic (Chapter 5).

Neoliberalism is not only confined to the exercise of state-to-state interactions. It has also extended into multilateral financial institutions such as the World Bank, the International Monetary Fund (IMF) and the Organisation for Economic Co-operation and Development (OECD) where Core countries have been exercising control over lending policies that align with neoliberal principles. The manifestations of neoliberalism in these institutions are the conditions that they set, called structural adjustment programmes or 'good governance' in academic jargon. These programmes include the adoption of liberal trade and investment, the rule of law, anti-corruption measures, higher taxes, and lower public spending, among others. As practice has shown,[24] in general, the effectiveness of these programmes is mixed, depending on various factors, including the local conditions of the recipient countries, timing, and the implementation process.

Neoliberalism in the US began in earnest under Ronald Reagan, carried on through George Bush, rose to its height during Bill Clinton, maintained itself through George Bush Jr., and declined during Barack Obama. Donald Trump pushed the American order to the far right, and Joe Biden restored a more centrist position by steadily increasing state input to the country's economic order using industrial policy. Neoliberalism is said to have ended with Obama, but remnants and legacies of neoliberalism have remained strong.[25] Its impacts have continued to be felt in the West and around the world.

THE STRUCTURE OF GLOBAL HEALTH

Global public health aims to improve the quality of life for everyone and so bring about health equality among people. If we accept the *global* nature of health – that we all share the same boat of well-being in this world – then it would be easier for us to accept the idea of health equity. Anything less would probably mean we accept differences in health outcomes among different people, which can be tolerated or, worse, ignored. This situation is, unfortunately (to many, but neutral perhaps to some), the reality of the world today.

The nature of international relations in general and international politics in particular renders the world in a situation of anarchy, a situation in which states – the main actors in world affairs – struggle among themselves for power. They interact with each other based on their calculation of interest and profit maximisation through the exercise of power and influence and through bargaining and negotiation. This reasoning by states permeates the global system, including that of the United Nations, wherein sovereignty rights are held high and treated as more or less sacrosanct. But the responsibility to protect public health lies first and foremost on the shoulders of individual states, and after that is meted out to inter-state cooperation. As such, health equity among all people becomes an ideal, an aspiration rather than a strict legal obligation, requiring states to do certain things, failing which punishments for non-compliance would apply. 'Health for all' or 'health equity' would then sound as hollow rhetoric or aspirational, representing a distant dream, elusive to many who need it to stay safe and alive.

This sorry state of affairs – disparity in global healthcare – has its origins and development very much in the process of colonialism and imperialism.[26] Colonisers from Europe (an assorted group of traders, soldiers and missionaries from various Christian countries in the region) explored Africa, America, and Asia. They did so to harness profits and interests from trade and extractive industries, protect overseas subjects and assets, and to find converts. The missionaries brought with them their medical knowledge to safeguard the health of their fellow traders and soldiers and, by extension, to promote and protect their collective interests. They also spent time learning about the diseases and illnesses that came from the colonies. The name of the London School of Hygiene & Tropical Medicine, now a high-ranking medical school forming a part of the University of London federation, bears some legacies of this colonial past. Founded in 1899 with a generous donation from an Indian philanthropist, it was established as a training ground to provide medical services to treat British colonial administrators and others working throughout Great Britain's tropical empire.[27]

Kew Gardens is another example with a strong link to the colonial past. Known also as the Royal Botanical Garden, it is located south-west of London. It reputedly houses the largest and most diverse collection of plant specimens from around the world. Opened in 1759, it has remained an important centre for conducting botanical science and horticulture. In its early years, British botanists and others from continental Europe would collect, smuggle, or steal plant specimens under exploitative conditions for political and commercial reasons,[28] with little or no regard for the livelihood of Indigenous peoples. In the process, forests were cleared, biodiversity destroyed, and the supplies of food and traditional herbal medicines disrupted. The ownership of many of the collected specimens (and seeds), some of which have been stored in Kew for centuries, has become controversial.[29] (More on Kew in Chapter 4.)

The asymmetric power relationship between the colonisers and the colonised in political, economic, social, and cultural life means that the ideas and institutions of Western medicine had the chance to be firmly established in the colonies while Indigenous medical ecologies were squeezed out. This kind of unbalanced relationship has now seeped through to become an unequal access to vaccination, as was displayed during the Covid-19 pandemic. While wealthy countries have hoarded large quantities of vaccines, many of which have been held past their expiration date, poor people in the Global South have been starved of vaccines and have suffered disproportionally from sickness and fatality. The system of intellectual property rights – patents and royalties – has been blamed for creating such a sorry state (more in Chapter 6).

SAME BED (STRUCTURE), DIFFERENT DREAMS (APPROACHES) (同床异梦)

Ngo Tak-Wing of the University of Macau, while reviewing China's style of globalisation using the BRI as a case study, identifies three distinctive features that set apart China's behaviour in international political economy from neoliberalism.[30] The first is that China's policy focuses very much on infrastructure building to make various kinds of connections, from physical and policy connections to trade, finance and cultural exchange, rather than on the production of any specific industrial or commercial goods in the global supply chain. The second feature is that China's approach is very state-centric. Chinese government agencies and state-owned enterprises are heavily involved in these infrastructure projects, rather than the multilateral corporations and private enterprises used in the neoliberal drive of contemporary global capitalism. And the third feature is that the nature of the risks involved are different between China's state-led model and the neoliberal model of the West.

Ana Cristina D. Alves of Singapore's S. Rajaratnam School of International Studies also cites infrastructure as the key feature of China's BRI. She points out that China's Belt and Road approach is pragmatic and flexible.[31] China sets few or no conditions on project cooperation, unlike the structural adjustments programme or good governance conditions set by Western countries, the World Bank, the IMF, and the OECD. China's pragmatism and flexibility are found in funding packages as well as in project implementation.

I have done a fair amount of analysis of the major characteristics of the BRI, identifying ten features of geo-developmentalism, a framework with which to study China's BRI. The evolving nature of the BRI necessitates a regular and close review of these features, something I will return to in the concluding chapter.

While the theoretical differences between the new geo-developmentalism and the well-established neoliberalism are quite clear, in practice there is a narrowing of the divide between the two approaches. While China continues to place strong emphasis on infrastructure connections, it has plans to make the projects more environmentally clean, less risky, smaller in size, and with a wider partnership. This includes the role played by the private sector, and even welcomes wealthy countries in the West to join forces in infrastructure building. The neoliberal countries led by the US and the EU are also changing, placing greater emphasis on infrastructure building and making greater use of industrial policy instruments such as state subsidies and strategic guidance. From an alternative perspective, the differences between the two are increasingly in degree rather than in kind.[32]

Despite the narrowing of the divide, some deep-seated differences have remained in place to hinder mutual accommodation, especially from the US perspective. One basic difference is their different ways of doing business. China uses a state-led approach to marshal resources with relative ease, bringing financial resources from major policy banks such as the Import-Export Bank of China and the China Development Bank to fund infrastructure projects. It can also marshal human resources like cheap labour from state-owned construction companies. The American way of doing business, however, is based very much on the free market. The government can work with private companies through private–public partnership, but the initiative and major contributions are sourced mainly from the private sector. In addition, Congress is very reluctant to pass legislation providing funding for huge infrastructure projects overseas. In response to China's BRI, the US has initiated programmes such as the Blue Dot Network, the Build Back Better Plan, and the Partnership for Global Infrastructure and Investment, with the US Agency for International Development serving as a coordinator. However, these initiatives are no match for China's sprawling BRI, in terms of funding, scale, and scope, according to a former American diplomat.[33] Apart from finance and economics, politics plays an important part: China is more attuned to the needs of partner countries in the Global South. It works with them rather than lecturing or directing them on how development should proceed.

CONCLUSION

Social inequality is clearly an indelible feature of the world today. The various aspects of this inequality are inter-linked, whether they relate to the consumption of food and water, the access to housing, education and medicine, or the ability to tackle climate change and population growth. All can be traced in one way or another to poverty as the ultimate source of human suffering, according to many observers and practitioners. The UN has identified the eradication of poverty as the primary goal of its Sustainable Development Goals. The way out of poverty is aid and development which are complementary to one another. In view of the aid fatigue experienced by many developed countries for various reasons including Covid-19, the war in Ukraine, and high inflation, it is largely up to developing countries to help themselves and assist each other. Here, China can offer help. Other emerging economies can help as well, through bilateral and multilateral methods and South–South cooperation, and the management and governance of the UN system. Against this background, the HSR is a welcome addition, as it forms one of the many instruments that can provide global assistance and development.

NOTES

1. From the aim and scope of *Global Public Health*, an international journal, https:// www .tandfonline .com/ action/ journalInformation ?show = aimsScope & journalCode=rgph20 (accessed 8 March 2023).
2. Solomon Benatar and Gillian Brock (eds), *Global health: ethical challenges*, 2nd ed. (Cambridge: Cambridge University Press, 2021), p. 1.
3. Paulo Afonso B. Duarte, Francisco José B. S. Leandro, and Enrique Martínez Galán (eds), *The Palgrave handbook of globalization with Chinese characteristics: the case of the Belt and Road Initiative* (Singapore: Springer Nature, 2023).
4. Barry Buzan, *An introduction to the English School of international relations* (Cambridge: Polity Press, 2014).
5. I did some preliminary analysis on the balance of power, the balance of production, and the balance of ideologies in world affairs and China's views; in Gerald Chan, *Chinese perspectives on international relations: a framework for analysis* (London: Macmillan; New York: St. Martin's Press, 1999), p. 184.
6. 'Capitalism', Wikipedia, https://en.wikipedia.org/wiki/Capitalism (accessed 19 September 2022).
7. 'What is capitalism: varieties, history, pros & cons, socialism', Investopedia, https://www .investopedia .com/ terms/ c/ capitalism .asp (accessed 19 September 2022).
8. 'What is capitalism', (accessed 21 August 2023).
9. Brett Christophers, *Rentier capitalism* (London: Verso Books, 2020); see also his *Our lives in their portfolios: why asset managers own the world* (London: Verso Books, 2023).
10. 'What is capitalism', IMF, https://www .imf .org/ en/ Publications/ fandd/ issues/ Series/Back-to-Basics/Capitalism (accessed 10 December 2023).
11. 'Capitalism vs. socialism: what's the difference?', Investopedia, https:// www .investopedia.com/ask/answers/020915/what-are-differences-between-capitalism -and-socialism.asp (accessed 19 September 2022).
12. Anton Malkin has co-authored an article on the use of extraterritorially by the US as a tool of structural power in the semiconductor industry and trade. See Anton Malkin and He Tian, 'The geoeconomics of global semiconductor value chains:

extraterritoriality and the US–China technology rivalry', *Review of International Political Economy*, 2023, https://doi.org/10.1080/09692290.2023.2245404.

13. 'Vatican formally rejects "Doctrine of Discovery" after Indigenous calls', PBS NewsHour (accessed 31 March 2023).

14. PBS NewsHour, 'Vatican formally rejects'.

15. Johan Galtung, 'A structural theory of imperialism', *Journal of Peace Research*, Vol. 8, No. 2 (1971), https://www.jstor.org/stable/422946 (accessed 6 January 2023). This paragraph is my interpretation of Galtung's work.

16. Hao Yun-p'ing, 'The compradors', in Maggie Keswick (ed.), *The thistle and the jade: a celebration of 175 years of Jardine Matheson* (London: Frances Lincoln Ltd., 2008), pp. 98–117.

17. See: https:// thedocs .worldbank .org/ en/ doc/ 20 6293abe6ad 06f4dc8c2f b541a3b93b -0330272022/ original/ Chancel2022WB .pdf (accessed 14 January 2023).

18. Barry Buzan, 'The "standard of civilisation" as an English School concept', *Millennium: Journal of International Studies*, Vol. 42, Issue 3 (2014), https://doi .org/10.1177/0305829814528265.

19. John King Fairbank, 'Ewo in history', in Keswick (ed.), *The thistle and the jade*, p. 287.

20. See: https://www.oecd.org/ctp/taxationcanpromoteequalitysaysinternationalt axdialogue.htm (accessed 12 June 2023).

21. A US Senate committee, however, voted in support of the 'Ending China's Developing Nation Status Act' in June 2023 to strip China of its status as a developing nation in some international organisations. China, of course, decries this act as unfair. See *China Daily*, Hong Kong ed., 31 July 2023, p. 15.

22. 'Neoliberalism', Wikipedia, https:// en .wikipedia .org/ wiki/ Neoliberalism (accessed 19 September 2022).

23. 'Neoliberalism', Investopedia, https://www.investopedia.com/terms/n/neoliberalism .asp (accessed 19 September 2022).

24. A good example is that of Indonesia under the IMF bailout during the Asian financial crisis of 1997–98. Malaysia, on the other hand, refused to accept IMF loan conditions and survived largely unscathed.

25. 'Book Review: The Rise and Fall of the Neoliberal Order', Australian Institute of International Affairs (accessed 14 April 2023), https://www.internationalaffairs .org.au/australianoutlook/book-review-the-rise-and-fall-of-the-neoliberal-order/

26. See: https://timesofindia.indiatimes.com/blogs/the-interviews-blog/global-health -has-its-origins-in-colonialism-and-imperialism-it-explains-why-iprs-are-used-to -withhold-technologies/ (accessed 11 April 2023).

27. 'London School of Hygiene & Tropical Medicine', Wikipedia, https:// en .wikipedia .org/ wiki/ London _School _of _Hygiene _and _Tropical _Medicine (accessed 11 April 2023).

28. See: https://www.plantsandculture.org/botanical-gardens-and-colonialism (accessed 21 August 2023).

29. BBC, 'Kew Gardens: botany and the British empire', https://www.bbc.co.uk/ programmes/w3ct5hzj (accessed 21 August 2023).

30. Ngo Tak-Wing, 'Foreword', in Duarte, Leandro, and Galán (eds), *The Palgrave handbook of globalization with Chinese characteristics*, pp. v–viii.

31. Ana Cristina D. Alves, 'BRI and global development praxis: is a paradigm shift eminent?', in Joseph Chinyong Liow, Liu Hong, and Gong Xue (eds), *Research*

handbook on the Belt and Road Initiative (Cheltenham, UK, and Northampton, MA, USA, 2022), pp. 81–83.

32. Gerald Chan, *China's digital Silk Road: setting standards, powering growth* (Cheltenham, UK, and Northampton, MA, USA, 2022), pp. 159–61.

33. Scot Marciel, 'Imperfect partners: The United States and Southeast Asia', webinar, East–West Center, Honolulu, 15 May 2023.

4.   China's health policy in Covid times

The new coronavirus that emerged in Wuhan in late 2019 has challenged the way we handle health prevention, preparedness, and response. The scale and speed with which the disease spread has seldom been seen since the Spanish flu a century ago or HIV/AIDS since 1980[1]: 2 million people died of Covid-19 worldwide in 2020, 3 million by April 2021, 4 million by July,[2] and 5 million by October.[3] On 11 March 2022, the BBC reported that 6 million people had died by the end of 2021. According to the British broadcaster, the figure could be as high as 18 million.[4] Although the death toll may have peaked in September 2022, WHO Director-General Tedros Adhanom Ghebreyesus warned that the pandemic was not yet over, as new variants might emerge to trigger more waves of disease in some countries.[5] In early May 2023, Ghebreyesus announced the end of the health emergency status of the virus.[6] The official death toll then stood at 7 million, although the figure could be three times as high.[7] He warned countries not to let down their guard; they should put their emphasis on the management of the disease and its long-term impact.

The Times of London says that sooner or later another major pandemic will appear.[8] Covid-19 has often been referred to as a 'once in a lifetime' or 'once in a century' pandemic, but scientists have estimated that another type of pandemic on a similar scale as Covid-19 has a 50 per cent chance of occurring in the next 25 years.[9] History has been punctuated by the emergence of such pathogens. The Black Death, for example, killed up to 200 million people in the 14th century. Russian or Asiatic flu, which scientists believe was likely to have been caused by a coronavirus, swept across the world in the 1890s, and is said to have taken a million lives. Spanish flu took 50 million lives in the aftermath of the First World War. In the past four decades, HIV has killed 40 million people. In recent decades, we have also experienced outbreaks of SARS, swine flu, MERS, Ebola, and Zika.

To draw lessons from the outbreaks of disease, this chapter provides a better understanding of what China has done to deal with Covid-19, both at home and abroad. What are the challenges the country faces? What has China done to tackle those challenges through its new health order, one in which the country is striving to strike a balance between using traditional Chinese medicine (TCM) and modern therapeutics? Above all, how has China emerged as one of the world's leading producers of medicinal drugs and medical equipment?

IS CHINA THE 'PHARMACY OF THE WORLD'?[10]

Many scientists around the world have laboured hard to produce the first drugs capable of containing the spread of the Covid-19 virus. The speed with which Chinese pharmaceutical companies have moved to mass produce vaccines to control the disease has taken many people by surprise. The mass production of drugs has revealed the extent to which the world's pharmaceutical industry is dependent on China for the supply of key ingredients used in making medicines.

Medicinal drugs are made from substances called active pharmaceutical ingredients (APIs). These ingredients are components designed to treat illnesses by, for example, suppressing a disease. They are responsible for the beneficial health effects experienced by consumers. An example of an API is the acetaminophen (also known as paracetamol) contained in a pain relief tablet.[11] In turn, APIs are made from substances called key starting materials (KSMs), which are usually rudimentary chemical substances making up the raw materials for APIs. As such, KSMs are the building blocks of APIs.

Up to the middle of the 1990s, the West and Japan had been producing about 90 per cent of the world's total amount of APIs. But in 2017 China alone produced some 40 per cent of all APIs.[12] It is now the top producer of APIs in the world. Such a phenomenal shift in global production of APIs is due partly to China's domestic demands and partly to its industrial policy for bringing about increased production. The ready availability of KSMs has lowered the cost of drug production. China has therefore enjoyed an advantage in the production of 'the low-cost and off-patent APIs' like antibiotics or vitamins.

India, a strong competitor in drug manufacturing, depends on China for its supply of APIs. Although India accounts for about 20 per cent of the global generic drug demand by volume, it imports about 70 per cent of its APIs from China.[13] While India is one of the biggest API exporters, many KSMs and other intermediate materials of these APIs are sourced from China. In the case of South America, Indian pharmaceutical companies have invested more in that continent than Chinese companies. Throughout the 21st century, Indian companies have consistently exported more finished pharmaceutical products to the region than Chinese companies. Yet, during the Covid-19 pandemic, it was China, not India, who supplied the majority of the region's vaccines.[14]

Several factors may have contributed to the rise of China's pharmaceutical industry.[15] First, the country led the world in the increase in filing of API patents between 2007 and 2021, followed by India, which also recorded an increase in filing during that period. Europe, Japan, Korea, and other countries, however, experienced declines in their filings. This situation gave China an enhanced income stream from patent revenues. Second, China's share of the production of APIs has grown rapidly, thanks to local and overseas demand and to the policy of the government to scale up the industry. Third, China is a big producer of generic drugs, which are much cheaper versions of branded products. Because of the rising costs of public health in almost every country, the use of generic drugs has become commonplace. In the US, for example, generics currently account for about 90 per cent of all prescribed drugs, up from 50 per cent in 2005. Although India is also a large producer of generics, China possesses an advantage because the cost of production in the country is 20 per cent lower due to easy access to KSMs and APIs. Fourth, China, like India, benefits from large-scale production.

Contrary to popular belief, China does not use only old-school methods for producing 'conventional' drugs, which utilise inactivated viruses to stimulate an immune response. It has also begun developing the new mRNA (messenger ribonucleic acid) drugs. The Chinese government aspires to become a great power in the pharma industry by naming bio-pharmaceuticals one of the ten industries to be nurtured as champion industries in its 'Made in China 2025' programme. As of November 2021, 20 Covid-19 vaccines from Chinese manufacturers were under clinical trial,[16] including both traditional and mRNA types – a tremendous effort rarely matched by other countries. (The new revolutionary mRNA vaccine trains the body's own cells to make a protein that triggers an immune response, without using any viral material. In the case of Covid-19, it produces a harmless piece of spike protein, stimulating the human body to defend itself against the virus.)[17] Although mRNA was first discovered and used as far back as the 1960s, it is Covid-19 that has encouraged its rapid development and widespread use, due in large part to commercialisation and government support.[18] At present, the US and some European countries are leading the development of mRNA technology, exploring possibilities of using such technology to treat other diseases including cancer.[19] As the immunity produced by vaccines wanes over time and new variants of viruses emerge, ongoing demands exist for the development of new vaccines to combat the new diseases. China's pharmaceuticals market is now only second in size to that of the US. The country aims to overtake the US in the near future and become the global leader in the pharma market.

The fact that the country has been a large producer of APIs for several decades and has increased its production of generic drugs more recently has helped China to become the largest exporter of Covid-19 vaccines. This has changed the global structure of the supply of pharmaceuticals. Five years ago, hardly anyone would have imagined that China could now export vaccines in such vast quantities.

China is not alone in catching up with the West in pharmaceutical production. Other countries in Asia are doing so as well, especially in the production of high-value drugs. As of 2021 all the top ten most profitable drug companies were in the US and Europe.[20] A year earlier two Asian countries were in the top ten (Takeda from Japan at No. 9, and Shanghai Pharmaceuticals from China at No. 10).[21] But countries like Thailand, South Korea, and Japan have been scaling up their vaccine development. Some of their companies have been partnering with Western firms under compulsory licensing agreements to produce Western branded drugs for sale at a lower price.[22] (More discussions on compulsory licensing in Chapter 6.)

In a series of reports published between late 2021 and early 2022 examining China's ascendance in vaccine manufacturing, *Nikkei Asia* of Japan cited three factors that have contributed to the rise of China as the 'pharmacy of the world'.[23] They are, in short: policy, people, and cash. China's human resources derive from locally trained personnel as well as those who have returned to China from overseas armed with knowledge and experience in pharmaceutical research, commerce, and regulations. In addition to government financial support, investments from private equities and venture capitalists in China's pharmaceutical sector have reached a record high – US$2 billion in 2021.[24] People and money aside, government policies have played an important role in providing an architecture to support the development of the bio-pharmaceutical industry. Table 4.1 shows major milestones in policy development since 2015 when China adopted its 'Made in China 2025' programme. The programme includes an advanced pharmaceutical industry as one of its ten key industries to be nurtured with a view to their becoming global leaders in their respective fields.

THE RISE OF CHINA'S MEDICAL DEVICE INDUSTRY

China's pharmaceutical industry has been growing rapidly. It is now the second-largest market in this sector of the world after the US, worth US$110 billion in 2017 and US$134.6 billion in 2018. Its size is expected to grow to US$161.8 billion by 2023, representing 30 per cent of the global market,[25] and to US$300.9 billion by 2025, growing at a compound annual rate of 12.2 per cent.[26]

Expanding side by side with its drug manufacturing is the country's medical device industry. A medical device can be understood as an instrument with a medical purpose. The WHO offers a more elaborate definition: 'a medical device can be any instrument, apparatus, implement, machine, appliance, implant, reagent for in-vitro (in-glass) use, software, material or other similar or related article, intended by the manufacturer to be used, alone or in combination, for a medical purpose'.[27] The world body has counted some 2 million kinds of medical devices on the world market, which can be categorised into 7000 generic device groups.[28] These devices include medical masks, medical protective gowns, ventilators and respirators, infrared thermometers, testing

Table 4.1   China's policies to promote the biopharma industry,
2015–2020

Year	Policy	Goals
2015	'Made in China 2025'	To develop biopharma as a key industry – one of ten industries
	Opinions on Reforming Review and Approval Process for Drugs and Medical Devices	To streamline approval processes
2016	Priority Review	To quickly assess innovative drugs and urgent treatments
	'Healthy China 2030'	To lay out a long-term plan to encourage innovation
2017	National Reimbursement Drugs List	To include innovative drugs
	Joining the International Council for Harmonisation of Technical Requirements for Pharmaceuticals for Human Use	To harmonise domestic standards with international ones
2018	60-day review rule	To facilitate clinical trial applications
	Volume Based Procurement	To open bids for central procurement of drugs and devices, raising quality, and lowering prices
2019	Drug Administration Law	To improve health legislation
	Marketing Authorisation Holder	To expand the scope of applications for drug market licences to R&D institutions and researchers, in addition to enterprises
2020	New Drug Regulation Registration	To clarify evaluation channels
	Patent Law	To institute a patent linkage system*

Note: * See Chapter 6 for details.
Sources: Adapted from 'China's global vaccine gambit', *Nikkei Asia*, Part 2: Pharmacy of the world, 23 December 2021, https://asia.nikkei.com/static/vdata/infographics/chinavaccine-2/ (accessed 26 May 2022); other internet materials.

reagents, precision medicine, wearable devices, and so on. Their purposes usually fall within one or more of four categories: prevention, diagnosis, treatment, or rehabilitation.

The Chinese medical device industry is already big, and it is growing bigger. In 2019 the industry registered revenues of 629 billion RMB, rising from 308 billion RMB four years earlier.[29] At an annual growth rate of around 20 per cent since 2015, the revenue figure climbed to over 800 billion RMB ($130 billion)[30] in 2020 and then to US$140 billion in 2021.[31] The industry has been growing more steadily in recent years at around 10 per cent per annum,[32] outpacing the country's GDP growth rate. As of 2019, medical equipment made up nearly 57 per cent of the medical device market, followed by high-end consumables (20 per cent), low-value consumables (12 per cent), and in-vitro diagnostics (11 per cent).[33]

At present, China accounts for about 20 per cent of the global medical device market.[34] This market share is estimated to grow at a compound annual rate of around 6 per cent[35] to reach 25 per cent by 2030 at US$218 billion. That would be second only to the US at US$300 billion. As of 2019, the US was far ahead of the world in the total medical device market, taking up 42.7 per cent of the global total, far ahead of second-place Japan at 7.2 per cent, third-place Germany at 7.1 per cent, and fourth-place China at 6.8 per cent.[36] In the same year, US suppliers captured 28.5 per cent of China's medical device imports, valued at US$5.46 billion.[37]

As a large developing country in rapid transition, China's medical device industry has been focusing mainly on the production of low-value products while importing high-value products from abroad. At present, China imports over 70 per cent of its medical devices.[38] However, the country has an ambitious plan to quickly upgrade the quality of its products and to substitute imports of high-value products with local ones. Several factors seem to have played a part in driving this change[39]:

- An ageing population with a rising disposable income;
- An increasing awareness of the need to achieve a high standard of hygiene and well-being;
- A gradual shift from disease treatment to disease prevention and health services;
- The proliferation of healthcare clinics and hospitals; and
- The low premiums on generic drugs, pushing Chinese pharma companies to look for alternative sources of income.

About 90 per cent of the domestic manufacturers of medical devices in China are small- to medium-sized businesses with capacity centred around producing low-value consumables such as disposable items and medical dressings. In the first half of 2021, the number of medical device companies in the country totalled 27 496, an increase from 13 000 in 2008.[40] (By comparison, the US had only 908 such companies in 2022.[41] But of course quantity and quality are two different matters.) A handful of foreign brands dominate the high-value medical device market in China, with the country importing around 70 per cent of high-value products such as diagnostic and therapeutic equipment. These multinational brands include Medtronic (US), General Electric (US), Siemens (US–Germany), and Philips (Netherlands). All four are among the top ten medical device companies in the world in 2022 in terms of total revenue.[42] At present, there are four Chinese companies in the top 100 medical multinationals, but none in the top 50.[43] The country is, however, working hard to catch up.

Its 'Made in China 2025' plan aims to produce 50 per cent of mid- to high-end medical devices by 2020, increasing to 70 per cent by 2025 and then 95 per cent by 2030.[44] This is to be achieved through the effective use of industrial policies that would include government subsidies and technology transfer.

HARMONISING MEDICAL REGULATIONS

As shown in Table 4.1, China comes very late to regulating medical products, let alone to harmonising its regulations with those of other countries. Covid-19 is a case in point. China was the first country to massively export its new coronavirus products to South-East Asia, including face masks, personal protective equipment, drugs, vaccines, respiratory ventilators, and other medical devices. The fact that South-East Asian countries have been following the medical standards and regulations of the United States and Japan means that Chinese shipments of these products have become relatively more expensive due to regulatory costs and long delays in usage approval.[45] This cost is multiplied to all concerned when facing a pandemic crisis. If China and the South-East Asian countries could increase the harmonisation of their regulations and standards, they would speed up the distribution of Chinese medical products and save lives. A similar situation applies to China's relations with other countries beyond South-East Asia. This is an area in which China needs to work harder and quickly in order to smooth the flow of its medical trade.

In terms of domestic institutional development, the establishment of the National Medical Products Administration (NMPA) is of great significance, as it serves a vital role similar to many comparable institutions in other countries, such as the Food and Drug Administration of the US. It was founded in 2018 to replace the former State Food and Drug Administration. In 2013 the former regulatory body was rebranded and restructured as the China Food and Drug Administration, elevating it to a ministerial-level agency. The NMPA is now a vice-ministerial-level administrative agency under the State Administration for Market Regulation.[46] It is responsible for creating and supervising the implementation of policies, plans, and standards governing the quality and safety of drugs, medical devices, and cosmetics. In addition, it oversees the post-market inspection of risk management and registration of licensed pharmacists. Unlike most other food and drug administrations around the world, the NMPA also has a rather unique role in looking after the regulation and promotion of TCM.

TRADITIONAL CHINESE MEDICINE

What is TCM? It refers to the medical practice that has been used for 3000 years in China. Based in large part on herbal treatment, it is usually administered by a publicly recognised professional who is knowledgeable in herbal medicines and their effects on patients. Within Chinese society, such practice is known simply as Chinese medicine. The adjective 'traditional' is, more often than not, used by people outside of China to make a clear distinction between it and Western medicine. The earliest written work of TCM is called *Huang Di nei jing* (黄帝内经 or *Yellow Emperor's Inner Canon*), compiled during the Warring States period (475–221 BCE).[47] It is a combination of philosophy, medicine, and religion, and its influence on Chinese medicine spanned more than 2000 years.

Western medicine is, of course, widely used around the world, including in China. It was introduced to the Qing China in the 19th century by missionaries from Europe. The use of TCM is, however, still very popular among ordinary Chinese, in mainland China as well as in overseas Chinese communities, because of tradition, availability, and low cost. This is so, especially among the elderly and people living in remote (rural) parts of China, where Western medical services are not easily available.

In contrast to Western medicine, TCM focuses much more on a holistic approach to treating the human body rather than on a specific part of it. TCM also focuses on balancing the functioning of various organs in the body rather than on symptoms in specific parts of the body. It aims at a longer-term treatment, rather than a quick fix. In a way, it is regarded by some practitioners as a way of life,[48] born out of Chinese culture and permeated into Chinese medical thinking. The concept of balancing extends from the human body to the relationship among humans to that between humans and nature as a way to live and work in harmony with the surrounding environment. The idea has also been extended to breathing exercises such as *qigong* (气功)and the practice of *tai-chi* or *taiqi* (太极, a smooth flowing, mild form of balancing movements) and even to more physically strenuous martial arts or boxing as a way to keep the body sound, both physically and mentally.

As an herbal treatment, TCM depends very much on plants and their ingredients and derivatives (also animal parts and to a lesser extent, things such as snake venom, rhino horns, deer antlers, and tiger bones). According to one count, there are some 368 000 plant species on our planet, and only about 40 000 of them are being used for making medicines, cosmetics, and functional supplements.[49] Western drugs are made using plant ingredients, and China has been the main supplier of many of these ingredients to pharmaceutical manufacturing companies in the West and in India. Interestingly, American trade sanctions on Chinese products do not seem to have covered these ingredients.

Herbal medicines have also been used in many other societies and cultures,[50] but it is in China that they have been extensively and intensively used over a very long period of time. China has been increasingly keen to promote TCM and to cooperate with other countries in developing herbal medicines.

Acupuncture has already been used to relieve pain in many parts of the world. Massage or *tuina* (推拿), in various forms, has been applied in many cultures, old and new. Moxibustion (the burning of herbal leaves on or near the body) and cupping (the use of warmed glass jars to create suction on certain points of the body) have become recognised practices for maintaining well-being. In the main, though, TCM has a long way to go to gain greater traction beyond China and the Chinese diaspora, due partly to the uncertain supply of quality plants, partly to the lack of convincing clinical evidence, and the lack of standardisation, among other reasons.

The Chinese government and many professional practitioners of TCM have been keen to promote the awareness and use of TCM around the world. One prominent development is the establishment of the World Federation of Chinese Medicine Societies in Beijing in 2003. The federation aims to promote international exchange and the dissemination and development of TCM. Established as a non-governmental organisation, it brought together at its inauguration 100 000 TCM practitioners from 100 societies in 44 countries.[51] Those coming from the US included delegates of the American Association of Oriental Medicine, the National Association of Chinese Medicine, the American Association of Chinese Medicine & Acupuncture, and the National Federation of Chinese TCM Organisations.[52] As of December 2021, the federation had 277 group members and 203 branches in 72 countries and regions.[53] It is affiliated with the WHO, the International Organization for Standardization, UNESCO, and the UN Economic and Social Council.

The WHO has recently begun to promote greater awareness of traditional medicines, including TCM. The global body has defined traditional medicine as 'the knowledge, skill and practices based on the theories, beliefs and experiences indigenous to different cultures, whether explicable or not, used in the maintenance of health as well as the prevention, diagnosis, improvement or treatment of physical and mental illness'.[54] In a report published in 2019, it has identified 98 of its member states as having developed national policies on traditional and complementary medicine (T&CM), 109 as having launched national laws or regulations on T&CM, and 124 as having implemented regulations on herbal medicines.[55] Many of these countries are in Asia and Africa. In the same report, the WHO has pointed out that 88 per cent of its member states have acknowledged the use of T&CM, corresponding to 170 member states.[56] In April 2022 the WHO set up its Global Centre for Traditional Medicine in Gujarati on the west coast of India to study, develop, and harness the values of traditional medicine.[57] In March 2023, the University of Macau announced that a permanent secretariat of the Western Pacific Regional Forum for the Harmonization of Herbal Medicines would be set up in the university to coordinate regional cooperation and to help develop the traditional medicine industry in Macau, a special administrative region of China like Hong Kong.[58]

A significant milestone in global health development is the inclusion of T&CM in a new chapter (Chapter 26)[59] in the latest, 11th, revision of the International Classification of Diseases (ICD-11) published by the WHO. The ICD grew out of the recognition of the need to compile such information among the fraternity of the medical profession in the West. The first classification system was adopted in 1893, based on a system developed by French statistician and demographer, Jacques Bertillon.[60] In the following years, it was known as the International List of Causes of Death and eventually as the ICD. Since its foundation in 1948, the WHO has assumed responsibility for publishing and revising the ICD, roughly once every ten years. In the 1980s and early 1990s, it had significantly revised the ICD, completing ICD-10 in 1990. The latest ICD-11 was adopted at the World Health Assembly in May 2019 and went into effect in February 2022.[61] This ICD contains a description of all known diseases and injuries in about 17 000 unique codes for injuries, diseases, and causes of death. These codes are underpinned by more than 120 000 codable terms. By using code combinations, more than 1.6 million clinical situations can now be coded, according to the WHO.[62]

The ICD works basically as a 'common language' that allows health professionals in Western medical systems to share health information across the globe. With the addition of traditional medicines in Chapter 26, a gaping hole in the global medical systems began to be filled. This may lead eventually to some integration of medical systems that would benefit all. At present, traditional medicines are largely developed independently in silos in various countries with little sharing of information, harmonisation, or standardisation. Chapter 26 has heralded a new change of direction in medical development, to the betterment of all.

In Europe, practitioners, educators, and supporters of TCM from Austria, Belgium, Germany, Ireland, the Netherlands, Sweden, and the UK have worked to create a united vision for the development, education, and standardisation of TCM. In April 2003, the European Register of Organisations of Traditional Chinese Medicine was officially recognised as an international non-profit corporation. Its 39 member associations came from 14 countries on the continent.[63]

In the UK, the Federation of Traditional Chinese Medicine Practitioners was established in 2002. It aims to achieve legal status in Britain for the Chinese medical profession. The Association of Traditional Chinese Medicine and Acupuncture is one of the self-regulatory bodies that govern TCM in the UK. The Chinese Academy of Medical Sciences Oxford Institute is China's first medical sciences institute in the UK, hosted by the University of Oxford. It is a collaboration between the Chinese Academy of Medical Sciences and the university. Kew Gardens, the Royal Botanic Gardens in south-west London, is noted for its huge collection of plant species from around the world. Since

1998, it has worked with the Institute of Medicinal Plant Development in China to collect some 700 plant species from various parts of China.[64]

In 2015 there were 3966 TCM hospitals in China, including 253 hospitals of ethnic minority medicine and 446 hospitals of integrated Chinese and Western medicines.[65] In addition, there were 42 528 TCM clinics. Put in context, there were 36 570 hospitals in the country in 2021, about two-thirds of which were privately owned.[66] China has great plans to expand the reach of TCM. At the fifth Belt and Road Forum for TCM Development held in Beijing in September 2022, Yu Wenming, the head of the National Administration of Traditional Chinese Medicine, said that TCM had evolved into a significant field for international collaboration, covering 196 countries and regions.[67] In the 14th Five-Year Plan period (2021–25), the Chinese government aims to jointly establish 30 high-quality TCM centres with countries along the Belt and Road. A TCM centre was first established in St. Petersburg, Russia, in 2016. Shortly thereafter, another was set up in Nur-Sultan, the capital of Kazakhstan.[68] More have been set up in major cities in subsequent years, including Barcelona, Budapest, and Dubai, totalling some two dozen by 2018.[69]

According to one analysis,[70] TCM products have been exported to about 163 countries around the world. TCM herbal medicine export reached almost US$1.2 billion in 2007, a rise of 8 per cent from 2006.[71] In 2021 the total export value of TCM products reached US$5 billion.[72] Depending on different definitions and calculations, Chinese herbal medicine represents 20–50 per cent of the herbal medicine market share worldwide.

These developments, though expanding, seem to represent thus far a relatively small advancement on the fringes of the overall development of the mainstream medical science in the world.

CONCLUSION

Covid-19 has put China in the limelight of global public health. The country has become one of the major providers of global healthcare. This happened very quickly, and China's achievements so far are by no means small, despite controversies and debates surrounding the origins of the virus and its handling of the fight against the virus, including the zero-Covid policy. It has become a major manufacturer of vaccines, medical supplies, and medical devices. It aspires to become a superpower in the global pharmaceutical industry. In the meantime, the standardisation and harmonisation of its medical standards with those of other countries are the major tasks facing the country going forward.

NOTES

1. The Spanish flu is said to have killed 50 million people, and HIV/AIDS 40 million.
2. See: https://www.who.int/emergencies/diseases/novel-coronavirus-2019 (accessed 8 July 2021).
3. See: https://www.stuff.co.nz/national/health/coronavirus/300442145/a-world-remembers-memorials-honour-covid19s-5-million-dead (accessed 2 November 2021).
4. See: https://www.bbc.com/news/health-60690251 (accessed 11 March 2022).
5. See: https://news.un.org/en/story/2022/09/1126621 (accessed 21 September 2022).
6. BBC World News, 6 May 2023.
7. 'Lockdowns not only cure for Covid', *Weekend Herald*, Auckland, 7 May 2022, p. A21.
8. Reprinted in *Weekend Herald*, 25 March 2023, pp. A12–A13. This paragraph is drawn from this source.
9. See: https://www.cgdev.org/blog/the-next-pandemic-could-come-soon-and-be-deadlier (accessed 6 May 2023).
10. This phrase is borrowed from 'China's global vaccine gambit', *Nikkei Asia*, Part 2: Pharmacy of the world, 23 December 2021, https://asia.nikkei.com/static/vdata/infographics/chinavaccine-2/ (accessed 29 August 2023).
11. See: https://www.canada.ca/en/health-canada/services/drugs-health-products/compliance-enforcement/information-health-product/drugs/active-pharmaceutical-ingredients-questions-answers.html (accessed 5 January 2023).
12. 'China's global vaccine gambit', *Nikkei Asia*, Part 3: The great medicines migration, 5 April 2022, https://asia.nikkei.com/static/vdata/infographics/chinavaccine-3/ (accessed 26 May 2022).
13. 'China's global vaccine gambit', 5 April 2022.
14. See: https://thediplomat.com/2022/05/india-vs-china-in-latin-america-competing-actors-or-in-separate-leagues/ (accessed 27 May 2022).
15. 'China's global vaccine gambit', 5 April 2022.
16. 'China's global vaccine gambit', 23 December 2021. For up-to-date tracking, see the database of the Vaccine Centre of the London School of Hygiene & Tropical Medicine, https://vac-lshtm.shinyapps.io/ncov_vaccine_landscape/ (accessed 13 June 2022).
17. 'WHO reveals countries to produce first COVID-busting mRNA vaccines in Africa', *United Nations News*, 18 February 2022, https://news.un.org/en/story/2022/02/1112212 (accessed 11 December 2023).
18. See: https://publichealth.jhu.edu/2021/the-long-history-of-mrna-vaccines#:~:text=Messenger%20RNA%2C%20or%20mRNA%2C%20was,to%20be%20brought%20to%20market%3F (accessed 10 June 2023).
19. See: https://www.ncbi.nlm.nih.gov/pmc/articles/PMC9647423/ and https://www.genengnews.com/topics/drug-discovery/rna-therapies-diversify-and-become-more-impactful/ (accessed 13 June 2023).
20. See: https://pharmaboardroom.com/articles/top-10-global-pharma-companies-2021/ (accessed 29 May 2022).
21. See: https://www.beckershospitalreview.com/pharmacy/top-10-pharma-companies-by-revenue-in-2020.html (accessed 29 May 2022).

22.   Hannah Elyse Sworn, 'COVID-19 is reshaping global pharmaceutical competition – to Asia's benefit', *The Diplomat*, 8 October 2021, https://thediplomat .com/ 2021/ 10/ covid -19 -is -reshaping -global -pharmaceutical -competition -to -asias-benefit/ (accessed 11 December 2023).
23.   'China's global vaccine gambit', 23 December 2021.
24.   'China's global vaccine gambit', 23 December 2021.
25.   See: https://daxueconsulting.com/pharmaceutical-industry-china/#:~:text=China's %20pharmaceutical%20market%20has%20been,86.4%25%20of%20total%20drug %20expenditure. (accessed 14 May 2022).
26.   See: https:// www .european pharmaceut icalreview .com/ news/ 156869/ chinese -patent-reforms-to-bolster-pharma-innovation/#:~:text=Patent%20reforms%20by %20China%20following,by%202025%2C%20growing%20at%20a (accessed 14 May 2022).
27.   See: https://www.who.int/health-topics/medical-devices#tab=tab_1 (accessed 30 November 2022).
28.   See: https://www.who.int/health-topics/medical-devices#tab=tab_1 (accessed 30 November 2022).
29.   'Chinese medical device industry: how to thrive in an increasingly competitive market?', Deloitte, 2021, p. 1.
30.   See: https:// www .amcham -shanghai .org/ en/ article/ insight -magazine -look -chinas-medical-devices-market-mncs (accessed 30 November 2022).
31.   See: https:// asia .nikkei .com/ Business/ Companies/ China -moves -to -shut -out -foreign-medical-equipment-makers (accessed 1 December 2022).
32.   'Chinese medical device industry: how to thrive in an increasingly competitive market?', p. 3.
33.   'Chinese medical device industry', p. 1.
34.   'Chinese medical device industry', p. 1.
35.   'China's focus to develop domestic medical device industry may discourage multinational companies', 27 September 2022, https:// www .globaldata .com (accessed 30 November 2022).
36.   See: https://www.khidi.or.kr/board?menuId=MENU01253 (accessed 30 November 2022).
37.   'Healthcare, China – country commercial guide', International Trade Administration, US Department of Commerce, https://www.trade.gov/country -commercial-guides/china-healthcare (accessed 20 December 2022).
38.   'What China's domestic agenda means for foreign medical device developers', Medical Device Network, 14 October 2022, https://www.medicaldevice-network .com/features/what-chinas-domestic-agenda-means-for-foreign-medical-device -developers/?cf-view (accessed 11 December 2023).
39.   'Chinese medical device industry', p. 2.
40.   'Number of medical device manufacturers in China 2008-H1 2021', https:// www .statista .com/ statistics/ 1076323/ china -medical -device -company -number/ (accessed 21 November 2022).
41.   See: https://www.ibisworld.com/industry-statistics/number-of-businesses/medical -device-manufacturing-united-states/#:~:text=There%20are%20908%20Medical %20Device,increase%20of%200.6%25%20from%202021 (accessed 3 December 2022).
42.   See: https://www.breakingintodevice.com/en-nz/blogs/medical-sales/top-medical -device-2022 (accessed 1 December 2022).
43.   'What China's domestic agenda means for foreign medical device developers'.

44. 'Chinese medical device industry', p. 4.
45. 'E-Commerce can help harmonize medical device standards and build China-ASEAN ties', https://www.globalasia.org/v17no1/cover/e-commerce-can -help -harmonize -medical -device -standards -and -build -china -asean -ties _anyu -leefujian-li (accessed 7 October 2022).
46. See: https:// chinameddevice .com/ faq/ general -questions/; see also the official website: https://www.nmpa.gov.cn/ (both accessed 5 January 2023).
47. See: https://en.unesco.org/silkroad/silk-road-themes/documentary-heritage/ (accessed 9 March 2023).
48. *China Report*, Beijing, October 2022, p. 49.
49. *China Report*, Beijing, October 2022, p. 49.
50. This includes, in the case of New Zealand, the Indigenous Māori traditional medicines made from indigenous plants and trees and the bones of whales.
51. See: https:// www .acupuncturetoday .com/ mpacms/ at/ article .php ?id = 28344 (accessed 11 October 2022).
52. See: https:// www .acupuncturetoday .com/ mpacms/ at/ article .php ?id = 28344 (accessed 11 October 2022).
53. See: http://www.wfcms.org/en/list/3.html (accessed 11 October 2022).
54. *WHO global report on traditional and complementary medicine 2019* (Geneva: World Health Organisation, 2019), p. 8.
55. *WHO global report on traditional and complementary medicine 2019*, p. 5.
56. *WHO global report on traditional and complementary medicine 2019*, p. 10.
57. See: https://www.france24.com/en/live-news/20220419-who-launches-traditional -medicine -hub -in -india (accessed 2 April 2023); 'WHO establishes the Global Centre for Traditional Medicine in India', WHO, https://www.who.int/news/item/ 25 -03 -2022 -who -establishes -the -global -centre -for -traditional -medicine -in -india (accessed 14 June 2023).
58. See: https://www.um.edu.mo/news-and-press-releases/press-release/detail/55207/ (accessed 2 April 2023).
59. An online copy of the ICD-11 can be found at 'ICD-11 for Mortality and Morbidity Statistics', https:// icd.who.int/browse11/l-m/en#/http%3a%2f%2fid .who.int%2ficd%2fentity%2f718687701 (accessed 27 December 2022).
60. International Classification of Diseases, *Britannica* (accessed 26 December 2022).
61. PAHO/WHO, 'WHO's new International Classification of Diseases (ICD-11) comes into effect', https:// www .paho .org/ en/ news/ 11 -2 -2022 -whos -new -international -classification-diseases-icd-11-comes-effect (accessed 27 December 2022).
62. PAHO/WHO, 'WHO's new International Classification of Diseases'.
63. See: https://www.acupuncturetoday.com/mpacms/at/article.php?id=28344.
64. See: https://www.acupuncturetoday.com/mpacms/at/article.php?id=28344.
65. *WHO global report on traditional and complementary medicine 2019*, p. 64.
66. See: https://www.statista.com/statistics/624593/china-hospital-number-by-ownership/ (accessed 10 March 2023).
67. 'TCM gains popularity among Belt and Road countries', *Xinhua*, https://english .news.cn/20220904/1bb129e1185442eb8aae623ebf10c7b0/c.html (accessed 13 October 2022).
68. 'TCM gains popularity'.
69. See: https:// www .nature .com/ articles/ d41586 -018 -06782 -7 (accessed 2 April 2023).

70. See: https:// www .ncbi .nlm .nih .gov/ pmc/ articles/ PMC7114631/ (accessed 5 April 2023).

71. For some data in earlier periods of China's export of medicinal products and the development of Chinese medicine, see, respectively, *The industrial map of China pharmaceuticals, 2006–2007* (in Chinese) (Beijing: Social Sciences Academic Press, 2006); and Meng Qingyun (ed.), *Zhongguo zhongyiyao fazhan wushinian (1949–1999)* [*Fifty years of development of Chinese medicine (1949–1999)*] (Zhengzhou: Henan Medical University Press, 1999).

72. See: https://www.statista.com/statistics/1231881/china-import-and-export-value -of-traditional-chinese-medicine/ (accessed 14 June 2023).

5. China's vaccine diplomacy and health governance

China is a newcomer to vaccine diplomacy – the use of vaccines as a means to achieve diplomatic goals or the practice of distributing vaccines abroad for diplomatic gains. The country is not known for exporting large quantities of vaccines until very recently. In January 2020, it started to sell small amounts of Covid-19 vaccines.[1] In 2021, it became the largest exporter of such vaccines.

Covid vaccines have attracted global attention in combating the spread of the virus.[2] What is a vaccine in the first place? In layman's terms, it is a biological substance designed to protect humans from infectious diseases.[3] It is a medicine that stimulates the body's immune system to fight against a virus it has not come into contact with before. Vaccines are administered to a human body to prevent a disease from attacking, rather than to treat a disease once a person has caught it.[4]

This chapter traces the rise of China's vaccine production and export. The country has been extending medical assistance to Africa since the 1960s, a continent that has suffered disproportionally from epidemics in the past. The continent is presently being ravaged by the Covid-19 pandemic due to a lack of vaccines or vaccination. Compared with other continents, the total mortality figure is low, however, because of speedy action taken to deal with the pandemic, a young population, and a warmer climate.[5] How has China conducted its vaccine diplomacy in Africa? How has the country engaged with global health governance? The chapter begins by tracking the origins and development of vaccines before discussing China's manufacturing of vaccines and their export to Africa and elsewhere.

VACCINES AND DIPLOMACY: ORIGINS AND DEVELOPMENT

The first inoculation or injection of a vaccine into a human body – through nasal insufflation or inhalation – took place in China in the 15th century.[6] The practice spread to other parts of Asia and Africa before reaching Europe in the 18th century. With the rise of global trade and the expansion of empires, smallpox began to ravage communities around the world.[7] In the early 18th century, in Europe alone this disease was estimated to have killed 400 000 people every year during the height of the pandemic.[8] The vaccine for smallpox, introduced by British doctor Edward Jenner in 1796, was the first successful vaccine to be developed in the West.[9] Within 20 years of its discovery, Jenner's vaccine was said to have saved millions of lives. Soon, smallpox vaccination had become a common treatment around the world. In 1980, the World Health Assembly declared the complete eradication of the disease. No cases of naturally occurring smallpox have been found since.[10]

In 1881, French biologist Louis Pasteur developed a successful vaccine against anthrax. Four years later he developed another vaccine, this one against rabies. In the 1960s, vaccines were developed for measles, mumps, and other diseases. At present, there are some 20 kinds of vaccines for diseases, including those for treating influenza and hepatitis A & B.[11]

The use of vaccines as a diplomatic tool has a long history, probably as long as the development of modern vaccines itself. British physician Edward Jenner might have been the first vaccine diplomat. His professional work was so well respected in Europe that he was regarded as an unofficial ambassador between warring states on the continent. When Jenner requested the French to release British prisoners of war, Napoleon Bonaparte was noted to have said, 'Jenner! Ah, we can refuse nothing to that man'.[12]

Throughout the 19th century, France distributed Louis Pasteur's rabies vaccines around the world with few border restrictions.[13] Nowadays, vaccines have been used by state authorities to promote public health domestically and internationally, to protect national interests, and to assert political influence, either by donating vaccines to countries in need, by selling them at a low price or, at the other extreme, by simply denying their access. Global vaccine diplomacy has seen a new light during the Covid-19 pandemic, in part because China engaged actively *for the first time* with a seemingly generous global distribution of vaccines. The country, of course, is not alone in doing this. India and Russia have also done something similar, as have the US and the EU,[14] all competing for soft power influence, image building, image repair, and market branding and promotion.[15] International organisations such as the WHO and UNICEF (the UN Children's Fund) are seen to be conducting such diplomacy for the common good.

MODERN VACCINES COMING TO CHINA[16]

In 1805, a Spanish physician named Francisco Javier de Balmis led a medical team to promote smallpox vaccination in the Spanish colonies. On his way home after finishing his trip to Manila, he stopped in Guangzhou where he set up smallpox vaccination stations. Subsequently, the Jennerian vaccination methods gradually replaced the traditional kind of inoculation used in China. A significant import from the West was the idea of a modern public health system. The earliest modern public health organisations in China were established by Westerners in the concession areas of treaty ports. Towards the end of a plague outbreak in north-east China in 1911, the Chinese government came to realise the importance of establishing a public health system. In 1919, the ruling Beiyang government (北洋政府, the government of the Republic of China, which sat in its capital Beijing between 1912 and 1928) established the Central Epidemic Prevention Bureau in Beijing, the first centralised government agency responsible for the prevention and treatment of infectious diseases. (In comparison, France established its central public health agency in 1822, Britain in 1850, the State of Massachusetts in 1850, and New York City in 1866.)[17] The bureau produced vaccines for various infectious diseases including cholera, typhus fever, dysentery, plague, and rabies. At that time, vaccines were produced and distributed in extremely limited amounts and vaccination was restricted to only a few big cities. In 1929, the Nanjing Government invited the League of Nations to send a health delegation to visit more than ten Chinese cities and towns, to inspect the healthcare situation and offer suggestions for improvement.[18]

During the war against Japan in the 1930s and 1940s, the bureau relocated to the south-western city of Kunming. Under its direction and with international assistance, Kunming became an important base for vaccine research and production. When the surrounding Yunnan province experienced a cholera outbreak, Kunming officials worked to publicise the importance of being vaccinated, sending medical teams to promote vaccination in urban areas and villages.

Three years after the founding of the People's Republic of China (PRC) in 1949, the central government launched a nationwide Patriotic Health Campaign to popularise vaccination as a way to prevent infectious diseases. In the 1960s, the creation of an extensive network of grassroots medical stations and the large-scale recruitment of so-called 'barefoot doctors' – individuals given basic medical training and sent to treat rural residents – led to a rapid rise in vaccination rates. In the first three decades of the PRC, infectious diseases such as cholera, tuberculosis, and diphtheria were effectively brought under control. In 1979, the country officially declared that it had eradicated smallpox.

CHINESE VACCINES TO COMBAT COVID-19

As seen above, compared with the West, China came relatively late to the use of modern vaccines. For example, the Chinese Society for Immunology, a voluntary non-governmental organisation (NGO), was only established in 1988.[19] However, Chinese pharmaceutical companies were among the first in the world to develop vaccines for combating Covid-19 in early 2020. In May 2021 the WHO granted Emergency Use Listing to Sinopharm, a vaccine produced

Table 5.1   *Total supply of vaccines by type, 31 May 2022*

Vaccine	No. of doses (millions)	Share	Cumulative share
AstraZeneca	3465.6	22.9%	22.9%
Sinovac	3165.3	20.9%	43.8%
Pfizer	3097.7	20.4%	64.2%
Sinopharm	2851.8	18.8%	83.0%
Moderna	1045.2	6.9%	89.9%
Johnson & Johnson	878.2	5.8%	95.7%
Sputnik V	310.1	2.0%	97.8%
Others	339.1	2.2%	100.0%

Source: WTO–IMF Vaccine Trade Tracker, https://www.wto.org/spanish/tratop_s/covid19_s/vaccine_trade_tracker_s.htm (accessed 10 October 2022).

in Beijing, paving the way for its inclusion in COVAX, a campaign organised by the WHO and other healthcare organisations to distribute Covid-19 vaccines and other medicines to poor countries.[20] A month later, Sinovac, another Chinese vaccine, was enlisted. This listing has helped to boost the global use of Chinese vaccines around the world. It has been estimated that in 2021, nearly half of the total doses of Covid vaccines produced worldwide was sourced from Chinese manufacture, either in factories on the Chinese mainland or based overseas.[21] In May 2022, CanSinoBIO became the third Chinese Covid vaccine to be listed, bringing the number of global vaccines so listed at that time to nine – Pfizer-BioNTech, AstraZeneca, Janssen, Moderna, Sinopharm, Sinovac, Bharat Biotech, Novavax, and CanSinoBIO. The listing of Russia's Sputnik V vaccine was stalled, due to Russia's invasion of Ukraine in February 2022.[22] As of May 2022, other vaccines in the process of being listed include another Sinopharm jab, produced in Wuhan, and vaccines from France's Sanofi, China's Clover and Zhifei Longcom, and Iran's Shifa Pharmed. Hundreds of candidate vaccines were being worked on in laboratories around the world, including 156 in clinical development (i.e. tested on humans) and 198 in pre-clinical phases.[23] How did the supply of Chinese vaccines compare with other supplies?

AstraZeneca, a vaccine designed with the help of scientists from Oxford University, was one of the first vaccines to be distributed around the world. In a promotion drive, the university stated that the vaccine 'made available 3 billion doses to more than 180 countries during the pandemic and has been judged to have saved 6.3 million lives during 2021'.[24] Table 5.1 shows a list of popular vaccines that have been used around the world, in comparison with AstraZeneca.

China is among the few countries in the world that can largely meet home demand for immunisation with locally produced vaccines. By the end of 2020, the country had granted approval to 55 vaccines for preventing 35 infectious diseases. Forty-seven domestic vaccines with lot releases were produced by 38 domestic companies in China. The number of doses of lot releases of domestic human vaccines came to 651 million in 2020. In the same year the total output value of human vaccines in the country was more than 60 billion RMB.[25] As of November 2021, China had provided more than 1.8 billion doses of Covid-19 vaccines to more than 110 countries and international organisations,[26] including 50 African countries and the African Union Commission,[27] UN peacekeepers, and the International Olympic Committee (for use in the Tokyo Games in 2020). The tally increased to 2.2 billion doses to over 120 countries and international organisations, as of June 2022.[28] At the same time, China cooperated with over 12 countries to produce or trial Covid-19 vaccines,[29] most of which are in Africa (Table 5.2).

Starting in December 2020, China became the first country to bulk export Covid vaccines to developing countries. At the same time, it was poised to become a major drug manufacturer in the world. Excepting China and India, the lack of vaccines has been plaguing many developing countries. Poverty and difficult access to medicines are the two major sources of poor health outcomes, affecting who bears the brunt of epidemics, the scourge of war, natural disasters, and the destruction brought about by climate change. Developing countries experience 70 per cent of the world's disease burden while taking up only 15 per cent of global health spending.

Across sub-Saharan Africa, one child in 13 dies before the age of five, compared to one in 200 for wealthy countries.[30]

Africa is the least vaccinated continent for Covid-19 on a per-capita basis: 7 per cent fully vaccinated compared with 28 per cent in lower-middle-income countries as of mid-December 2021.[31] According to the UN Development Programme, as of 27 July 2022, only one in five people or 21 per cent in low income countries have been vaccinated with at least one dose, whereas the corresponding figure for high-income countries is three in four or 72 per cent.[32] By January 2022, 9 billion Covid vaccine doses had been produced worldwide, but only 540 million of them found their way to Africa. This is 6 per cent of all Covid vaccines, despite the continent's 16.7 per cent of the world's population.[33] The continent has administered 309 million doses, so that less than 10 per cent of Africans are fully vaccinated. In other words, approximately 1.2 billion Africans have not yet received a single jab. At the January 2022 rate, much of the continent may not be vaccinated until 2023.[34]

Africa's call for help has not gone unheeded, however. A growing number of governments, development finance institutions, foundations, and public–private entities have offered assistance.[35] As of March 2021, GAVI (the Global

Alliance for Vaccines and Immunisation) and UNICEF provided finance and procurement of approximately two-thirds of the total market value of vaccines in Africa.[36] About 70 per cent of the volume procured for GAVI-supported countries originated in India, but only 30 per cent of the value.[37] In April 2021, the WHO made an open call for help in launching an mRNA vaccine technology transfer hub in South Africa.[38] (More on mRNA later in this chapter and the next.) In June 2021, leaders of the Group of Seven wealthy countries agreed to support 'African efforts to establish regional manufacturing hubs'.[39]

Many Western countries have made significant contributions to Africa or have pledged to do so, including France, Germany, the UK, Canada, and the US. Beyond the West, China, India, and Russia have made contributions as well. The United States had belatedly, in an announcement made by President Joe Biden in September 2021, pledged to donate over a billion Covid-19 vaccine doses for global use. Its International Development Finance Corporation and partner institutions have plans to invest in vaccine production in Senegal and South Africa.

Foundations and philanthropists such as the Bill and Melinda Gates Foundation, the MasterCard Foundation, the Jack Ma Foundation, and others have also chipped in to help. Financial institutions like the African Development Bank, the World Bank, WHO, Coalition for Epidemic Preparedness Innovations (CEPI), UNICEF, GAVI, and others have contributed in one way or another. In late May 2022, Pfizer, the top pharma earner in the world by a huge margin, proposed 'An Accord for a Healthier World' to close the health equity gap for 1.2 billion people living in 45 lower-income countries.[40] In January 2023, Pfizer announced that it would expand its initial offerings of vaccines and medicines from 23 to 500 products.[41]

The global distribution of medical aid is complex. In most cases, the entities involved engage in a hub-and-spokes mechanism to expedite the flow of assistance in regulation and procurement. In the case of Africa, six major hubs (countries) for vaccine manufacture have been identified by the African Union and the African Centres for Disease Control and Prevention. They are Egypt and Tunisia in the north of the continent, South Africa, Ethiopia to the east, Senegal to the west, and Rwanda in the middle. China has been actively involved in the manufacture and distribution of drugs in many of these hubs. It has also been involved in technology transfer and capacity building, especially in Addis Ababa, the capital of Ethiopia,[42] from where Chinese medical supplies are distributed to neighbouring countries and on to the rest of the continent.

A LONG AND WINDING (SILK) ROAD TO AFRICA

Modern China has been relatively late in reaching out to Africa. However, 600 years ago during the Ming Dynasty (1368–1644), Chinese navigator and diplomat Zheng He, in his seven major ocean voyages, sailed his majestic fleet across the South China Sea and the Indian Ocean to reach the east coast of Africa. The voyage along this (old) maritime Silk Road was, however, short-lived, as it was cut short by the Ming emperor.[43]

Earlier, China had intermittent contacts with the African continent through trade and migration, dating back many centuries and spanning a number of ancient dynasties. Historians and archaeologists have differing views as to when China established its first contact. Li Anshan, a specialist on overseas Chinese in Africa at Peking University, has pointed out that it could have been as early as 138–126 BCE (prior to the Qin Dynasty, 221–206 BCE).[44]

According to a seasoned Chinese observer,[45] it was the Portuguese sailors, under the captaincy of explorer Vasco da Gama, who arrived on Africa's west coast in 1418. From then on, Africa was connected with the modern world (meaning Europe). The continent became the target of colonial exploitation and enslavement by European powers. By 1914, with the exception of Ethiopia, nearly all parts of Africa had been carved up by European colonisers. After the Second World War, African countries gained their independence one after another. The Europeans left behind an economic vacuum to be filled by Indian and Pakistani traders. The mining of gold in Africa attracted prospectors from many corners of the world, including 64 000 Chinese who went to South Africa between 1904 and 1910.[46] The number of Chinese nationals working in Africa peaked at 263 659 in 2015 but dropped sharply to 104 074 in 2020,[47] because of travel bans due to Covid-19. The pandemic has slowed down the progress of many BRI projects which employ large numbers of Chinese labourers.

In a report on China's engagement with Africa, *The Economist* of London points out that the contemporary history of China–Africa relationships has three phases.[48] During the Cold War, the first phase, China supplied aid, constructed the odd railway or parliament building, and tried, with little success, to implant Maoism. The relationship in this phase was largely political, with China wooing the newly independent states in the continent, winning their support to vote China into the UN and replace Taiwan in 1971. The second phase, from the 1990s onwards, was largely defined by economics. China imported oil and minerals from Africa. In return, the country extended aid and investments. The election of Xi Jinping as China's top leader in 2012 started the third phase, in which China has doubled down on its political and economic investments in the continent. This has alarmed the West – the US and the EU in particular. The modern Silk Roads, under the umbrella of the BRI, launched by Xi in 2013, have reached wide and deep into Africa.

In response to China's BRI, the US proposed the Build Back Better World (B3W) under the Biden administration in 2021. This was followed shortly by the EU's Global Gateway. At the G7 summit held in Germany in June

2022, the leaders agreed to launch the Partnership for Global Infrastructure and Investment (PGII) to strengthen partnerships with developing countries through the building of environmentally greener and politically cleaner projects, coalescing the B3W and the Global Gateway. At the following G20 summit held in November 2022 in Bali, Indonesia, the G7 countries reaffirmed their commitment to launch the PGII, pledging to mobilise US$600 billion for global infrastructure investment by 2027. The US has pledged US$200 billion and the EU €300 billion.[49] An observer has pointed out that the PGII would face two major tests in the near future: one is how to attract private investors to join; the other is how to create an integrative process so that the whole partnership would be greater than the sum of its individual parts or projects.[50] Another observer has pointed out that the pledged amount of US$600 billion (even if it is new money and forthcoming), spread evenly over five years, is unlikely to make any huge impact on the trending shift of OECD aid funds from economic and productive sectors to domestic administrative costs and refugee spending (on Ukrainian refugees in Europe).[51]

China's medical aid to Africa has gone through the above-mentioned three phases of development with little interruption. In fact, the country has intensified its activities under the HSR during Covid times. The assistance package consists of[52]:

1. The dispatch of medical teams;
2. The building of hospitals and medical infrastructure;
3. The donation of drugs and medical equipment;
4. The training of healthcare workers; and
5. The control and prevention of infectious diseases such as malaria and Ebola and, more recently, Covid-19.

Of these five areas, the dispatch of medical teams has been seen as the flagship of China's medical assistance. Under Maoist revolutionary zeal to help the Third World, China sent a medical team to Algeria in 1963, despite experiencing abject poverty at home, to show solidarity with Africa in the fight against colonialism, imperialism, and hegemonism. Subsequently, help was extended to Somalia, Congo Brazzaville, Mali, Mauritania, and Guinea during the 1960s.[53] Up to September 2022, China had dispatched medical teams consisting of more than 28 000 professionals to 73 countries, providing basic healthcare for over 290 million patient visits, according to *China Daily*.[54] At the end of 2021, around 1000 Chinese medical workers worked in 45 countries in Africa.[55] Some of them also helped combat Covid-19. The primary task of these medical teams was to provide services and training to the local community and to build the health capacity of the host country. Each province of China has been 'twinned' with one or more host countries for arranging the dispatch of appropriate personnel. Some 45 hospitals in 40 African countries are paired in this way.[56] Normally each medical team would consist of clinicians, nurses, a leader, a translator, and a chef. Team size varies from half a dozen people to a hundred. The average tour of duty ranges from one to two years.

According to Ammar A. Malik, a researcher at the AidData programme of the College of William & Mary in Virginia, China's commitments to the world in the health sector from 2000 to 2017 included 1448 projects costing a total of US$5.6 billion. Most of them are in Africa: 1047 projects worth US$2.7 billion.[57]

The Eighth Ministerial Conference of the Forum on China–Africa Cooperation (FOCAC), held in Dakar, Senegal, in November 2021, presents a good opportunity to take stock of the state of the bilateral relationship between China and Africa. China has been Africa's largest trading partner since 2009. It is the continent's biggest source of foreign direct investment, surpassing the US in 2013.[58] Numerous infrastructure projects have now been completed; others are ongoing. These projects involve the building of roads, bridges, railways, airports, seaports, power plants, hospitals, telecommunication stations, and many more. China and African countries have agreed to work closely together on nine programmes: healthcare, poverty reduction and agriculture, trade promotion, investment, digital innovation, green development, capacity building, people-to-people exchanges, and peace and security.[59] Many of these programmes are in line with China's BRI objectives. Both parties aim to start implementing these nine programmes in the first three years (2021–23) of their China–Africa Cooperation Vision 2035 plan.[60] The plan, formulated at the FOCAC conference, paves the way for future strategic partnerships to 2035 with a view to improve the quality of their joint projects.

Under the healthcare programme, China aims to assist the African Union in achieving the latter's goal of vaccinating 70 per cent of the African population against Covid-19 by 2022. To help achieve this goal, President Xi Jinping pledged to provide another billion doses of vaccines to Africa, in addition to the 200 million doses that had already been delivered.[61] Of these 1 billion doses, 600 million would be donated and 400 million would be co-produced on the continent by Chinese pharmaceutical companies and their African counterparts. China has also undertaken to build ten medical and health projects for African countries and send 1500 medical personnel and health experts.[62]

A landmark project is the construction of a new headquarters for the Africa Centre for Disease Control and Prevention in Addis Ababa, fully funded by China and agreed upon at the FOCAC summit held in Beijing in 2018. The topping-out ceremony of the headquarters building was held in November 2021. Phase one of the construction was completed in January 2023, with the newly appointed Chinese Foreign Minister Qin Gang (suddenly deposed in July 2023) joining the officiating ceremonies.[63] The project is scheduled for completion by the end of 2023.[64] In 2012, China helped build the African Union's headquarters, also in Addis Ababa, at a cost of US$200 million. In December 2022, China signed an agreement to build a headquarters for ECOWAS (Economic Community of West African States) in Abuja, Nigeria, at a cost of US$31.6 million.[65] Due for completion in February 2024, it would house the ECOWAS Commission, the Community Court of Justice, and the ECOWAS Parliament.

CHINA EXPORTING VACCINES TO AFRICA

The development of vaccines normally takes years to complete. In the case of Covid-19, however, major pharmaceutical companies around the world were competing with each other to develop the first vaccine, with strong financial backing from their respective governments. Moderna created its vaccine on 13 January 2020,[66] only two days after the genetic sequence of the virus was openly published by Chinese scientists.[67] Other vaccine developers followed in hot pursuit, including the Chinese.

China was the biggest exporter of Covid vaccines worldwide in 2021. Most of these exports were conducted through commercial deals. This is not surprising, considering the health security situation at a time when countries were competing with each other to get as many vaccines as possible and as soon as possible to protect their own citizens. Asian countries received the vast majority of Chinese vaccines for financial, cultural, and logistical reasons. Chinese global exports have started to drop off significantly since January 2022 as more vaccines with better efficiency have become available and as demands for vaccines have lessened[68] for various reasons: pandemic fatigue, vaccine hesitancy, complacency, and others.

Bridge Consulting in Beijing had compiled an online database to track Chinese exports of vaccines, giving an up-to-date and comprehensive picture of China's vaccine distributions,[69] up until the country ditched its zero-Covid policy in January 2023. As of 28 December 2022,[70] the consultancy said that China had sold 1.85 billion Covid vaccine doses and donated 328 million. The country had physically delivered 1.65 billion to over 100 countries, establishing itself as the largest exporter at the time. Many of the recipient countries have also received donations, sales, or pledges from the US and European countries. In terms of deliveries, the Asia-Pacific region has received the largest share of Chinese jabs, some 890 million doses, followed by Latin America (290 million), Africa (125 million), and then Europe (57.5 million to a few east European countries). China has also delivered 160 million doses to COVAX (a multilateral mechanism) for distribution to poor countries at low cost.

Before the start of its full-fledged vaccine diplomacy in April 2020, China began to distribute face masks and other personal protective equipment to countries in need, including developed countries, a move that has been referred to by observers as 'mask diplomacy'. Some see this Chinese move as returning a favour to others because China had received generous medical aid from other countries when it was suffering from the outbreak of Covid-19 earlier in the year. To others, these Chinese diplomatic activities were seen as an extension of China's soft power to repair its tarnished image over its initial (seemingly) clumsy handling of the outbreak of the virus in Wuhan in December 2019. The following events, in chronological order, mark the progress of China's vaccine exports[71]:

- In July 2020, the first Chinese vaccine (CoronaVac) trial outside China commenced in Brazil.
- In December 2020, the first batch of Sinovac vaccines was delivered to Indonesia and Turkey.
- In March 2021, India banned the export of its locally produced vaccines subsequent to a sudden spike in infection of the coronavirus in the country, which created a heavy demand for homemade vaccines. This led China to announce many pledges of donations and vaccine sales to countries like Indonesia, Brazil, Chile, and Mexico, creating the first peak in its vaccine deliveries.
- In June 2021, the WHO listed Sinopharm and Sinovac vaccines for emergency use, thus rolling out these Chinese vaccines for global use and leading to a sharp rise in Chinese vaccine exports.
- In July 2021, GAVI, the vaccine alliance, and other COVAX partners announced the signing of a deal to buy 550 million Chinese vaccines.
- In August 2021, at an international forum to discuss vaccine cooperation, President Xi Jinping pledged to provide 2 billion vaccine doses by the end of the year.
- In September 2021, China partnered with vaccine manufacturers in Egypt, Morocco, and other countries to boost local production in Africa.
- In October 2021, China's vaccine deliveries reached their highest point due to heavy demand overseas, in particular Iran which imported 86.3 million doses of Sinopharm.
- In January 2022, however, a significant drop in Chinese vaccine deliveries occurred due to several factors: the lifting of India's ban of its vaccine exports, thus boosting global supplies; the decline of global demand for vaccines; and the availability of Western vaccines with greater efficacies, such as Pfizer and Moderna, which had started to pick up distribution overseas in the second half of 2021.

China has by now provided vaccines directly to 118 countries around the world. The Asia-Pacific region has received the largest share of Chinese vaccines in 39 countries, followed by Latin America in 22 countries. In contrast, while Africa has 47 countries receiving Chinese vaccines, the continent has received fewer doses than Asia or South America. As a region, Europe has received the least number of Chinese vaccines. So far, ten European countries, mostly in the east, including Turkey, Bosnia and Herzegovina, Azerbaijan, Albania, and others, have received Chinese vaccines. In terms of actual deliveries, at the end of 2022, the top ten countries receiving the most Chinese vaccines were, in descending order of the number of doses: Indonesia (268 million), Iran, Pakistan, Brazil, the Philippines, Myanmar, Morocco, Mexico, Cambodia, and Vietnam (42 million).[72]

Throughout 2022, China's global export of vaccines remained flat, trickling to a tiny amount at the beginning of 2023. The country has shifted its focus from exporting to helping localise production in recipient countries and transferring technology to fight Covid-19 and future pandemics. This shift of focus could assist developing countries to independently produce vaccines, lessen their reliance on imports, and provide them with the opportunity to become a vaccine supplier to other low-income countries. Table 5.2 highlights some major activities of this new Chinese initiative.

Together, China's four major Covid vaccine developers (Sinovac, Sinopharm, CanSino, and Zhifei Longcom) have entered into 22 joint production agreements with various countries, as of March 2022 (Table 5.2). They have also recorded high sales and profits, although subject to wild fluctuations due to intense competition among manufacturers and the sharp rise and fall of global demands. In the first half of 2021, Sinovac reported sales revenue of US$11 billion, a 160-fold increase over 2020. CanSino reported a turnaround from a net loss to a net profit in 2021. Zhifei Longcom reported a net profit of 3.45 billion RMB in the first half of 2021.[73] The giant Sinopharm group reported an annual revenue of over 521 billion RMB for the full year of 2021.[74] Chinese companies are, however, no match for the world's top earner, Pfizer of the US, which reported a 92 per cent operational growth in revenue to a staggering US$81.3 billion in 2021, from US$41.7 billion in 2020.[75]

Pharmaceutical companies in the West have offered help in developing vaccines in some African countries. Some of these countries have also worked with Chinese manufacturers. For example, Pfizer and Moderna are building factories of their own, with early moves to South Africa, Rwanda, and Senegal.[76] South Africa's Biovac (established in 2003) has entered into agreements in July 2021 with Pfizer and BioNTech to produce up to 100 million doses of vaccines annually for exclusive use in Africa. On 1 March 2022, a consortium of nine development partners announced they would support Biovac expanding its existing vaccine manufacturing capacity.[77] The

Table 5.2   *China's vaccine tech transfer and joint productions, 2020–22*

Region	Country	Partners	Targets (No. of doses)
Africa	Algeria	Saidal | Sinovac	5 million per month starting from Jan 2022
	Egypt	Vacsera | Sinovac	1 billion per year; fully automatic fridge storage facility for 150 million
	Morocco	Sothema | Sinopharm	5 million per month
	Nigeria	Ongoing discussion	
Asia	Bangladesh	Incepta | Sinopharm	5 million per month
	Indonesia	Bio Farma | Sinovac	Regional production hub
		Etana Biotech | Abogen Biosci	100 million per year starting 2024 (mRNA)
	Malaysia	Pharmaniaga | Sinovac	Multiple goals
	Myanmar	Myancopharm | Sinopharm	5 million per month
	Pakistan	PakVac | CanSino	Cut price of locally produced vaccines
	Sri Lanka	Kelun | Sinovac	13 million initially
Middle East	United Arab Emirates	Hayat-Vax | Sinopharm	200 million per year
Central Asia	Uzbekistan	Jurabek | Zhifei Longcom	10 million per month
Europe	Hungary	National | Sinopharm	Develop medical infrastructure
	Serbia	Hemopharm | Sinopharm	3 million per month
	Turkey	| Sinovac	Cater in part for export, e.g. Libya
Eurasia	Russia	PetroVax | CanSino	From trial to production
Latin America	Argentina	| Sinopharm	
	Brazil	Butantan | Sinovac	100% local production
	Chile	| Sinovac	50 million per year
	Colombia	| Sinovac	Agreement signed
Central America	Mexico	Drugmex | CanSino	1.2 million per week

Note: Countries not in partnership with China include those of the 5 Eyes, Group of Seven, Quad, and AUKUS. This coincides with the sharp political divide between China and the West.
Sources: Bridge Consulting, Beijing.

goal is to increase production of pharmaceuticals locally in Africa to meet 70 per cent of local demand by 2030, and increase production of vaccines to 60 per cent by 2040.[78] These partners include the African Development Bank and development finance institutions from the UK, the US, and the EU.

A large number of Chinese public institutions and private companies have also been working with South Africa to combat Covid-19. These include the Bank of China, e-commerce giant Alibaba, and the Chinese diaspora in the country. Also involved are telecom giant Huawei, the Industrial Bank of China, China Construction Bank, and Land Pac, a construction company.[79]

Senegal in West Africa rolled out its vaccination programme using Sinopharm vaccines, then Oxford-AstraZeneca through COVAX.[80] The country has sent medical students to China to receive training. In June 2021, it signed a deal with a Belgian biotech group called Univercells to produce vaccines locally, starting in 2022. In this way, Senegal joins Egypt, Morocco, and South Africa in successfully securing rights to produce Covid vaccines.[81] The Pasteur Foundation in Dakar has experience in producing yellow fever vaccines since 1937. Morocco's pharmaceutical firm Sothema also works with China's Sinopharm to produce Covid vaccines. It also works with Sweden's Recipharm to produce Covid and other vaccines to meet the demands of the country and beyond.[82]

CHINESE BILLIONAIRES COMING TO THE RESCUE?

An intriguing feature of China's vaccine diplomacy is the active role played by privately–owned enterprises (POEs). The Jack Ma Foundation and the Alibaba Foundation have led the way for other Chinese POEs and NGOs to follow in helping countries around the world tackle Covid-19 with deliveries of much needed medical supplies. In March 2020, the two foundations donated over 1 million test kits and 600 000 face masks to African countries via Addis Ababa.[83] This was followed a month later by 500 ventilators and 200 000 personal protective gear kits.[84] In total, the foundations headed by Jack Ma delivered some 120 million face masks, 4.1 million test kits, 800 000 protective suits with masks, and 3704 ventilators to over 150 countries: 54 in Africa, 24 in Latin America, and many more in Asia and other places.[85] Other Chinese donors have followed suit, including tech giants Huawei and Tencent.

Chinese philanthropists have contributed large sums of money to research and development in the fight against Covid-19. As of mid-2020, the total contribution they made was estimated at 1.8 billion RMB (US$256 million).[86] Funders include the Jack Ma Foundation, Tencent Charity Foundation, Evergrande Group, Baidu, and others. Their donations largely supported Chinese research institutes and a few others in Australia, Italy, the US, and elsewhere.[87] By the end of 2018, the total charitable expenditure of Chinese foundations amounted to almost 6 billion RMB (US$0.86 billion).[88]

Chinese philanthropic gifts on such a large scale and at such a speed are unprecedented.[89] Clearly, the wealth of these philanthropists has grown enormously on the back of China's economic growth, especially in the last decade or so. China's *Blue Book of Philanthropy (2020)* says that the number of foundations (基金会) in the country soared from 3000 in 2012 to almost 8000 by the end of 2019.[90] Another reference, the *Annual Report on China's Philanthropy Development (2022)*, points out that there were 8885 foundations at the end of 2021, out of a total of 900 900 social organisations in the country, including 371 000 social groups and 521 000 social service institutions.[91] Most of the foundations are based in Beijing. They make grants and act in ways not dissimilar to foundations in other parts of the world. Some of them work more like NGOs while others, like GONGOs (government-organised NGOs).

The country has generated an economic environment that nurtures a large number of nouveau riches, especially in the tech sector and more recently the health sector. The 2021 Hurun Global Rich List, published in Shanghai, shows that there are 1058 billionaires in China and only 696 in America, increasing China's lead since 2019. The two countries have registered over half of the known billionaires in the world.[92] The top ten billionaires are mostly American, led for some time by Elon Musk,[93] the boss of Tesla, SpaceX, and Twitter. His crown was taken by Bernard Arnault, a French business tycoon and art collector, in December 2022.[94]

China's billionaire list is more volatile, for four reasons.[95] First, the rapid changes in the high-tech industry, chalking up some notable successes but also experiencing major setbacks. Second, the policy changes of the government which impact heavily on the fortunes of the rich. Third, the emergence of equity financing; and four, the country's shaky situation, in which stakeholders try to strike a balance between socialism and capitalism, between state and market, and between state-owned enterprises and private companies. Covid-19 and the war in Ukraine have affected the fortunes of many billionaires around the world – in China,[96] the US,[97] and elsewhere. Some have seen their fortunes evaporate, while others have continued to amass great wealth even during Covid times.

Of the 200 wealthiest individuals in China, over 46 have set up foundations.[98] The total amount of giving by Chinese philanthropies from 2009 to 2017 has averaged an annual increase of about 20 per cent.[99] The *Charity Law* (慈善法) of 2016 has provided a legal framework for charitable organisations to proliferate by clarifying what constitutes charitable status and by providing increased transparency and clarity as to the requirements of information disclosure by these organisations.

The *Charity Law* has stimulated the growth of charitable trusts in the country as well. By mid-2020, 415 charitable trusts had been established nationwide. Of these, 142 were established in the first half of 2020, with assets totalling 263 million RMB.[100] These trusts work to alleviate poverty, prevent and control epidemics, provide education, and pursue other charitable causes. Tackling the Covid-19 pandemic has recently become a priority for these trusts. An interesting feature of the development in charitable work in China is the popularity of online charity, thanks to the widespread use of internet technology and social media. According to an official of China's Ministry of Civil Affairs, in 2021 Chinese netizens donated nearly 10 billion RMB through online channels, up 18 per cent from the previous year.[101] The e-commercialisation of charity in China has become a new phenomenon in the evolving interface of technology and civil society in a cashless country.[102]

China's billionaire philanthropists have received much encouragement from the government to achieve 'common prosperity'[103] or, in essence, a more even (re)distribution of wealth among the general public. They have also received government pressure to do so, subtly or overtly.[104] On the whole, it appears that the private sector in China, including enterprises and social organisations, has overshadowed the government, central or local, in distributing aid overseas in tackling the global pandemic. To what extent will Chinese philanthropy make a difference in foreign aid in future? This would require continuing observation and analysis.

AFRICAN VACCINES FOR AFRICA: WHY, WHEN, AND HOW?

Africa is a continent of 54 countries and 1.4 billion people, 16.7 per cent of the world's population.[105] For decades, it has been producing less than one per cent of the vaccines that it consumes. The remaining 99 per cent have come mainly from the West and India through aid and procurement made by international agencies such as GAVI, a partnership representing international donors and pharmaceutical companies. This is secured at low prices, with UNICEF helping to distribute the vaccines to low- and middle-income countries through its well-established logistical network. Often placed by vaccine suppliers at the end of the queue, African countries have to endure the scourge of pandemics more than others. The continent has come under severe test by the ravaging Covid-19, a situation that it has vowed to change.

Despite lagging behind in vaccine development, Africa is not without its own drive. In 2007, the African Union adopted a plan called the 'Pharmaceutical Manufacturing Plan for Africa' to facilitate local pharmaceutical production. In 2010, a group of concerned Africans launched the African Vaccine Manufacturing Initiative to promote the establishment of sustainable vaccine manufacturing capacity in the continent so as to break the cycle of dependency on outside charity.[106] More recently, the African Union and the Africa CDC (Centres for Disease Control and Prevention) have spearheaded a continent-wide effort to combat Covid-19 and other diseases. The goal is for African countries to provide sufficient and affordable vaccines for Africans.

According to a report titled 'Partnerships for African vaccine manufacturing (PAVM) framework for action' published in early 2022, PAVM is designed 'to coordinate and enable partnerships within and between countries and with the global community of supporters'[107] to manufacture local vaccines. It aims to mobilise an investment of US$30 billion over the next 20 years: US$5 billion for capital expenditures and other one-off initial costs; and US$25 billion for funding recurring costs over a 20-year period. The bulk of the investments, about US$20 billion, would go towards supporting R&D.[108]

Established by the African Union in 2021, PAVM has an ambitious goal to develop, produce, and supply over 60 per cent of the total vaccine doses required on the continent by 2040,[109] a gigantic leap from around one per cent at present. The target is to lift the production volume to over 2.7 billion doses by 2040. By then, the public market for vaccines in Africa will have reached an estimated US$3 billion to US$6 billion, or even US$10 billion to US$17 billion if there is a sustained demand for vaccines.[110] In a bigger picture, the African pharmaceutical sector is expected to grow from US$19 billion in 2012 to US$66 billion by 2022 – the fastest such growth in the world.[111] The wider health and wellness sector is projected to reach US$259 billion by 2030.[112]

At present, only five countries in Africa can produce vaccines: Egypt, Morocco, Senegal, South Africa, and Tunisia. The African Union has identified six countries as having been engaged in talks with international partners to establish drug substance and fill-and-finish capacity in 12 production facilities. These six countries are Algeria, Ghana,[113] Morocco, Nigeria, Rwanda, and Uganda.[114] Of these, only Egypt, South Africa, and Algeria have plans to make Covid-19 vaccines from scratch.[115] Other countries in the continent with potential capabilities have been profiled for production.[116] Egypt stands out as the more advanced in making vaccines in the continent: its drug company Vacsera produced its first anti-venoms in 1881.[117] The country has become the first in Africa to produce Covid vaccines with the help of the Chinese Sinovac Biotech, which also helped build a high-tech cold storage system in the country. Completed in September 2022,[118] Egypt is poised to become a major distribution hub of vaccines in the northern part of the continent and to nearby areas of the Middle East.

Before 2020, nearly all international partners for vaccine manufacturing in Africa were Western companies. Thereafter, Chinese enterprises entered the African market to fill the missing gaps in the supply chain. Table 5.2 above shows some of these partnership arrangements. With outside help, can Africa undertake such a mammoth task of massively scaling up local production of vaccines? What are the obstacles standing in the way?

There are four major hurdles: one is the lack of investment to make things happen; second, the fragile health infrastructure on the continent; third, the lack of government commitments to buy locally produced vaccines; and fourth, the weak regulatory regimes in African countries struggling to meet international standards. Additionally, Africa faces such technical difficulties as the lack of cold storage facilities (to cater for its hot climate), efficient transport logistics, and an on-time supply chain of ingredients to make vaccines. Added to these difficulties are social impediments such as superstitions about health issues, ignorance and complacencies, hesitancies surrounding vaccination, and aid dependency.

In November 2021, South Africa's Aspen, the continent's largest pharmaceutical company, secured a deal to make Covid-19 vaccines under licence with Johnson & Johnson, an American pharma giant. Production started in early 2022. However, by April 2022, not a single order had been received from African customers. The precise reasons for this lack of interest are unclear. It could be because hundreds of millions of free doses had become available by then.[119] It could also be because of issues of pricing and financing, given the very tight budgets of many governments. This apparently disappointing outcome is likely to dampen African efforts to produce vaccines locally. For example, the WHO and its partners established the first Covid-19 mRNA vaccine technology transfer hub in South Africa in June of 2021.[120] The tech transfer from Western pharmaceutical companies has now been put on hold,[121] as Moderna plans to set up its first African mRNA vaccine manufacturing facility in Kenya. BioNTech also plans to set up its modular mRNA manufacturing facilities in Senegal, Rwanda, and South Africa. Egypt, on the other hand, is already producing Sinovac Covid-19 vaccines, having started since early 2022. Also in early 2022 the WHO added Bangladesh, Indonesia, Pakistan, Serbia, and Vietnam to the list of recipients of mRNA technology,[122] potentially creating more competitors in the world market.

In May 2022, African heads of state issued a statement urging GAVI, COVAX, and governments on the continent to prioritise purchases of vaccines from African plants, suggesting that they should commit to buying 30 per cent of the continent's output.[123] However, GAVI said that a lack of demand meant that it was 'not in a position to order large quantities of vaccines'.[124] In fact, in early December 2022, the GAVI board decided to scale down its vaccine purchases.[125] It was reported that GAVI had reached settlements with Moderna, the Serum Institute of India, and several Chinese manufacturers to cancel unneeded doses, surrendering US$700 million in prepayments in the process.[126] COVAX, on the other hand, may have exhausted its financial reserves. Thus, Aspen's fate as a Covid-19 vaccine producer hangs in the air. If African countries cannot pull themselves together to find a way out of this conundrum, they may find themselves unprepared when the next pandemic hits.

Meanwhile, instead of letting their production machines lie idle, Aspen entered into a deal with the Serum Institute in late August 2022 to produce four other vaccines under Aspen's brand name for sale and distribution in Africa. These four vaccines – hexavalent, pneumococcal, polyvalent meningococcal, and rotavirus – are commonly administered in Africa.[127]

ASSESSING CHINA'S VACCINE DIPLOMACY

Assessing China's vaccine diplomacy is by no means easy. Much depends on at least three variables: first, China's vaccine diplomacy is a relatively new undertaking, so any assessment at this point in time would be premature. Second, Covid-19 is continuously evolving, producing new variants and, hence, new waves of the disease could appear to change the calculus. Crisis behaviour and crisis management to deal with the virus are likely to remain typical of the responses of many stakeholders around the world, although some may be more prepared than others in facing the challenge. Third, vaccine manufacturing, sales, and distribution are more often than not shrouded in secrecy for commercial or security reasons. Such information is not easily available for public scrutiny. Added to these variables are the unintended consequences for global health development as a result of the politicisation of the issue in inter-state relations.

Given these complications, Wang Xiaoyi, a researcher of international trade and global health, has identified three distinctive features of China's Covid-19 vaccine landscape[128]:

1. Extensive Chinese partnerships in sales and manufacturing with low- and middle-income countries (see also Table 5.2);
2. Prioritisation of recipient countries that are associated with China's extensive BRI;
3. A nearly 50–50 split of investments by Chinese private and public sectors in R&D projects that produced Chinese vaccines. These investments totalled US$1 billion as of December 2021.[129]

CHINA ENGAGING GLOBAL HEALTH GOVERNANCE

In what way has China's vaccine diplomacy affected its engagement with global health governance? Here, global health governance is defined as the management of the protection and promotion of health for all at the global level. It is centred around (but not solely on) the activities of the WHO, a UN specialised agency set up in 1948 to promote global public health. China's participation in the activities of this organisation provides useful hints for gauging the country's contributions (or otherwise) to global health governance.

A year after its entry into the UN in 1971, China replaced Taiwan as a member of the World Health Assembly. Its initial contacts with the WHO were minimal. During the initial HIV/AIDS outbreak in the 1980s, China's (lack of) response to the pandemic and its own poor healthcare system was criticised by the WHO. It was not until the outbreak of SARS (severe acute respiratory syndrome) in 2002–03 did contacts between China and the WHO begin to increase. Relations with the WHO had become crucial for China to modernise its healthcare system.[130] Since then, the country has strengthened its engagement with the global health body in combating such infectious diseases as HIV/AIDS, avian flu, and swine flu. When Ebola erupted in 2014, China answered the WHO call for international help; it proactively sent medical teams and supplies to West Africa to deal with the outbreak.[131] This is a significant change to the nature of its foreign health assistance – from strictly bilateral to more multilateral. It has also played a more proactive role in engaging with various international and regional forums, such as the Global Fund to Fight AIDS, Tuberculosis, and Malaria; the ASEAN Plus Three (APT) Seminars on Enhancing Cooperation in the Field of Non-Traditional Security Issues; the International AIDS Conference; and the International Congress on AIDS in Asia and the Pacific. A special APT summit held in April 2020 adopted an 18-point resolution to deal with Covid-19, including the establishment of the Covid-19 ASEAN Response Fund for emergencies, the exchange of information, the setting up of reserves of essential medical supplies, and the training of public health workers, among others.[132]

China's contributions to the work of the WHO can be gauged using three measures: monetary contributions, personnel contributions, and policy inputs. The WHO derives its income from two main sources: assessed contributions and voluntary contributions. Assessed contributions are like membership fees calculated relative to a member state's wealth and population. These contributions make up less than 20 per cent of the WHO income. Voluntary contributions make up the other 80 per cent. These voluntary contributions are made by international organisations, philanthropic foundations, and the private sector, in addition to member states, to fund specific programmes or projects called for by the WHO. The top five member states making assessed contributions in 2022 are: US (US$109.3 million), China (US$57.4 million), Japan (US$41 million), Germany (US$29.1 million) and the UK (US$21.9 million).[133] The Trump administration slashed or withheld American contributions. As of June 2022, the assessed contribution of the US for 2022 was still listed as unpaid on the WHO website.[134] The Biden administration, however, has renewed its support for the WHO. Secretary of State Anthony Blinken said in early 2021 that the US would pay its membership fees owed.[135] The core voluntary contributions from member states come mainly from Europe, with the UK leading far ahead of others. In the 2020–21 biennial assessments of voluntary contributions, the top five contributors were the UK (US$135.13 million), Sweden

(US$35.79 million), Australia (US$32.56 million), the Netherlands (US$15.92 million), and Denmark (US$13.53 million).[136]

In April 2020, shortly after the Trump administration announced the freezing of its monetary contributions to the WHO, China pledged to contribute US$30 million to the organisation to help deal with Covid-19 and to strengthen the healthcare system of developing countries. This amount was in addition to a pledge of US$20 million made a month earlier for a similar purpose. Overall, in terms of monetary contributions to the WHO, starting from a low base which has remained relatively low compared with developed countries, China has been making significant monetary contributions to the WHO over the decades. Apart from the WHO, China has also provided US$50 million to the UN and other international organisations for dealing with the pandemic.[137]

In terms of policy contributions to the World Health Assembly, China has been playing low key agenda-setting and has shied away from debates and negotiations. This is so due partly to the lack of experience of its diplomats and delegates, partly to its generally low health system capacity at home, and partly to the country's long tradition of social and cultural practice – its diplomats generally do not feel comfortable with open debates in public forums. Like their participation in many other major international organisations (traditionally dominated by the West), Chinese diplomats have been on the whole rather timid and at times clumsy in their behaviour, apart from giving prepared speeches delivered in mandarin Chinese.

In terms of personnel contributions to the WHO, the 2006 election of Dr Margaret Chan, a former director of Hong Kong's Department of Health, to head the WHO marked a major improvement in bilateral relationships. Chan's top position in the organisation was a rare incidence. Although ethnically Chinese, she is a much more Western-trained and Western-minded Hongkonger compared with most mainland Chinese officials. Chinese nationals working in high-ranking positions at the WHO are few and far between. As of September 2022, the highest ranking Chinese national working in the WHO headquarters in Geneva is a medical doctor named Ren Minghui. He serves as Assistant Director-General for Universal Health Coverage/Communicable and Non-communicable Diseases.[138]

Participation in the activities of the WHO has provided valuable opportunities for Chinese representatives and delegates to learn more from the WHO about global health practice than for China to make significant policy inputs. China's major contributions to global health governance are, on the whole, very much based on offering practical and technical help to the developing world and on strengthening its healthcare system back home.

Indeed, China has a long-term plan to improve its healthcare system. The Healthy China 2030 vision, adopted in 2016, aims to achieve five goals by 2030: (1) improve the quality of health; (2) control major health risks; (3)

enhance health service capacity; (4) expand the scale of the health industry; and (5) streamline the health service system. According to the WHO, the Chinese government's health expenditure has increased more than threefold from 482 billion yuan in 2009, when health reform began, to 1640 billion yuan in 2018.[139] According to the State Council – the Chinese near equivalent of a government cabinet comparable to the West, the country's public health expenditure reached 1.9 trillion yuan (about US$293 billion) in 2020, a rise of 15.2 per cent over the previous year.[140]

In 2016, China and the WHO signed the China–WHO Country Cooperation Strategy (2016–2020) in Beijing, which is aimed at enhancing collaboration in health policies, planning, technology, and human resources. A year later the country signed a memorandum of understanding with the world body on the Implementation Plan on the Belt and Road Health Cooperation Mechanism. This MoU seeks to promote cooperation in health emergency response, prevention and treatment of infectious diseases, as well as in traditional medicine between countries along the Belt and Road.[141] (See Chapter 4 on the outreach of traditional Chinese medicine.)

The International Health Regulations (2005), which grew out of the response to deadly epidemics that once devastated Europe,[142] now form the legal basis of the work of the WHO. As an instrument of international law, the regulations are binding on 196 countries, including the 194 member states of the WHO. The regulations define the rights and obligations of countries in handling public health events and emergencies that have the potential to cross territorial borders. These include the requirement of states to report public health events. The regulations also outline the criteria to determine whether or not a particular event constitutes a 'public health emergency of international concern', events such as Covid-19, and more recently monkeypox.[143]

In 2021, the Ministry of Science and Technology of China signed an MoU with the CEPI to promote cooperation and exchange in the field of epidemic preparedness and innovation.[144] Launched at the World Economic Forum in Davos, Switzerland, in 2017, CEPI is a partnership among public, private, philanthropic, and civil organisations to develop vaccines to control various epidemics like Ebola and Rift Valley Fever. It worked with the WHO to deal with the emergence of Covid-19.

At the Asia and Pacific High-level Conference on Belt and Road Cooperation in June 2011, 29 countries, including China, launched the Initiative for Belt and Road Partnership on Covid-19 Vaccines Cooperation.[145] These countries work together in vaccine co-production, distribution, and mutual assistance.[146] Because of its efficient logistics and transport infrastructure built up over recent years, like the LOGINK platform,[147] China is in a good position to help transport medicines and medical equipment to the developing world and beyond. This has been demonstrated by China's massive deliveries of vaccines and personal protective equipment to various parts of the world in 2021.

China's relations with the International Council for Harmonisation of Technical Requirements for Pharmaceuticals for Human Use (ICH) are critically important to the country as it aspires to become a global leader in drug manufacturing. The ICH brings together regulatory authorities and the pharmaceutical industry to discuss scientific and technical aspects of pharmaceuticals and to develop guidelines for standardisation. Initiated in 1990, the ICH has a mission 'to achieve greater harmonisation worldwide to ensure that safe, effective and high-quality medicines are developed, and registered and maintained in the most resource efficient manner whilst meeting high standards'.[148] It held its inaugural Assembly in October 2015, establishing itself as an international legal entity under Swiss law. The founding members are the drug administration authorities of Europe, the US, and Japan. The association has grown to include 20 members and 36 observers (as of 2022). The WHO is one of its regular observers. China started to reform its drug review and approval system in 2015. Its drug regulatory authority, the National Medical Products Administration, joined the ICH as a regular member in 2017, and was elected a member of the ICH management committee in 2018.[149] Since then, China's drug registration administration system has accelerated its integration with international practices. It has transformed and implemented many ICH guidelines, as have a growing number of other national regulatory authorities.

To help developing countries achieve the UN Sustainable Development Goals (UNSDGs), China established in 2015 a South–South Cooperation Assistance Fund with a base capital of US$2 billion. This was increased to US$3 billion in 2017. At a BRICS summit held online in June 2022, President Xi Jinping pledged to add another US$1 billion to the fund and renamed it the Fund for Global Development and South–South Cooperation. President Xi also promised to increase funding to the UN Peace and Development Trust Fund. He said Covid-19 had eroded the gains in global development in the recent past and countries now faced new difficulties in realising the UNSDGs.[150] In September 2021, Xi floated the idea of a Global Development Initiative (GDI) in a video speech before the UN General Assembly to try to galvanise various efforts to achieve the UNSDGs. Initial responses from some developing countries and UN organisations have been positive (to be discussed in Chapter 8).

CONCLUSION

China's health diplomacy in general and its vaccine diplomacy in particular have largely been zooming in on the developing world, especially Africa. Developing countries have been more receptive of China's medical assistance for historical, ideological, political, and economic reasons.

Three interesting features have stood out from our examination of China's vaccine diplomacy: one is the role played by the private sector, largely in partnership with the government, in the R&D, production, export, and distribution of vaccines and medical supplies. The second is China's changing diplomatic focus from the export of Covid vaccines to their co-production with local manufacturers in host countries and to the building of their healthcare capacity, including the transfer of technology.[151] The third feature is China's preference to conduct such diplomacy in a bilateral way, although it has also increased its multilateral engagements to help enhance its national interests based on mutual benefits. These national interests include not only economic returns, but also the gaining of greater political influence as well as forging a better image of China as a responsible power in world affairs.

Despite Western bans and boycotts, China has managed to attract interested buyers and found suitable markets for its vaccines and other health products. Some of these markets have traditionally been dominated by the West. Before the rise of China and the outbreak of Covid, developing countries, including China, have had little choice but to purchase some of their medicines from the West at a high price, relying heavily on branded vaccines developed and produced by Western pharmaceutical companies.

History has shown that vaccine inequity has affected Africa badly, contributing in a significant way to the high rates of infection. Covid-19 has only confirmed this situation. The monopoly over the development of life-saving drugs, their manufacture, pricing, and distribution has been dressed up, rightly or wrongly, as the protection of patent rights, at least it is so perceived by the majority of the world's poor – a controversial topic we now turn to in the next chapter.

NOTES

1.   See: https://bridgebeijing.com/our-publications/our-publications-1/china-covid-19-vaccines-tracker/#Timeline_of_Vaccines_Delivered_by_China (accessed 22 November 2022).
2.   The word vaccine comes from the Latin *vaccinia* for cowpox.
3.   See: https:// www .winchesterhospital .org/ health -library/ article ?id = 222982 (accessed 21 May 2022).
4.   See: https://vk.ovg.ox.ac.uk/vk/how-do-vaccines-work (accessed 21 May 2022).
5.   See: https://gdc.unicef.org/resource/coronavirus-africa-five-reasons-why-covid-19-has-been-less-deadly-elsewhere (accessed 10 March 2023).
6.   'Variolation', Wikipedia, https://en.wikipedia.org/wiki/Variolation (accessed 7 June 2022).
7.   The old trade Silk Roads had served as conduits for the spread of diseases, medicines, and medical knowledge. UNESCO has published a series of articles on this. See https://es.unesco.org/silkroad/node/11065 (accessed 20 February 2023).

8. See: https://www.bbc.com/future/article/20200928-how-the-first-vaccine-was -born (accessed 3 June 2022).

9. Jenner might have learned his vaccine knowledge from the Indians or the Chinese through the Ottomans. See: https:// timesofindia .indiatimes .com/ blogs/ the -interviews -blog/ global -health -has -its -origins -in -colonialism -and -imperialism-it-explains-why-iprs-are-used-to-withhold-technologies/ (accessed 11 April 2023). See also Ou Jiezheng, *Dang zhongyi yushang xiyi* [*When Chinese medicine meets Western medicine*], rev edn (Hong Kong: Joint Publishing [H.K.] Co., Ltd., 2023), p. 78.

10. See: https://www.cdc.gov/smallpox/index.html#:~:text=Smallpox%20Virus& text=Thanks%20to%20the%20success%20of,occurring%20smallpox%20have %20happened%20since (accessed 29 May 2023).

11. See: https://www.reidhealth.org/blog/history-of-vaccines#_msocom_1 (accessed 3 June 2022); https://www.hhs.gov/immunization/diseases/index.html (accessed 15 June 2022).

12. See: https://www.nature.com/articles/144278a0 (accessed 4 June 2022).

13. See: https://www.csis.org/analysis/shot-heard-around-world (accessed 4 June 2022).

14. See: https:// ec .europa .eu/ commission/ presscorner/ detail/ en/ ip _21 _6283 (accessed 10 March 2023).

15. See: https://www .ncbi .nlm .nih .gov/ pmc/ articles/ PMC8259554/ (accessed 17 August 2022).

16. This section is sourced from Liu Xiaomeng, 'A brief history of Chinese vac- cination campaigns', 20 May 2021, https://www.sixthtone.com/news/1007516 (accessed 29 May 2023). For a detailed historical account, see Jiang Yonghong, *Zhongguo yimiao bainian, 1919–2019* [*One hundred years of Chinese vaccines, 1919–2019*] (Hong Kong: Kaifang shudian, 2021).

17. Jiang, *Zhongguo yimiao bainian*, pp. 23–4.

18. Ou, *Dang zhongyi yushang xiyi*, p. 107.

19. See: https://www.nature.com/articles/ni0408-339 (accessed 29 December 2022).

20. Founded in April 2020, COVAX is a global initiative to ensure fair access to Covid-19 vaccines worldwide. It is directed by the GAVI Vaccine Alliance, the Coalition for Epidemic Preparedness Innovations, and the WHO, together with UNICEF, a key delivery partner.

21. See: https://www.knowledgeportalia.org/vaccines-china (accessed 4 July 2022).

22. See: https:// www .pharmaceutical -technology .com/ news/ who -delays -sputnik -russia/ (accessed 13 August 2022). Other reasons may include the inconsistency in production in Russia.

23. 'WHO authorises CanSinoBIO Covid jab', *AFP*, 20 May 2022.

24. 'The Queen's anniversary prizes for higher and further education', a pamphlet distributed with *The Times*, London, 8 October 2022.

25. Huang Zhiming et al., 'Review on drug regulatory science promoting COVID-19 vaccine development in China', *Engineering*, No. 10 (2022), p. 128.

26. Zhiming et al., 2022, p. 128.

27. 'Xi announces supplying Africa with additional 1 bln COVID vaccine doses', *Qiushi* [*Seeking Truth*], 30 November 2021.

28. 'WHO pushes new COVID vaccine technologies', *China Daily*, internet ed., 22 July 2022. Former Prime Minister of Egypt: China has made an irreplaceable contribution to global solidarity against the epidemic (qq.com) (accessed 23 July 2022).

29. 'WHO pushes new COVID vaccine technologies'.
30. See: https:// www .aljazeera .com/ news/ 2022/ 5/ 25/ pfizer -to -offer -low -cost -medicines-vaccines-to-poor-nations (accessed 26 May 2022).
31. See: https:// www .nature .com/ articles/ d41591 -021 -00073 -x (accessed 7 June 2022).
32. *Human development report 2021/2022* (New York: UN Development Programme [UNDP], 2022), p. 6.
33. See: https://www.brookings.edu/blog/africa-in-focus/2022/01/24/vaccine-inequity -ensuring-africa-is-not-left-out/ (accessed 31 May 2022); https://www.worldometers .info/world-population/africa-population/ (accessed 1 May 2023).
34. See: https://www.brookings.edu/blog/africa-in-focus/2022/01/24/vaccine-inequity -ensuring-africa-is-not-left-out/ (accessed 31 May 2022); https://www.worldometers .info/world-population/africa-population/ (accessed 1 May 2023).
35. See: https:// www .interna tionalheal thpolicies .org/ featured -article/ a -synopsis -of -current-global-support-for-africas-vaccine-manufacturing-roadmap/ (accessed 26 May 2022).
36. 'Vaccine manufacturing in Africa', DCVMN member briefing – presentation document, UK Aid, 17 March 2021, p. 16.
37. 'Vaccine manufacturing in Africa', p. 17.
38. 'Establishment of a COVID-19 mRNA vaccine technology transfer hub to scale up global manufacturing', https://www.who.int/news-room/articles-detail/ establishment-of-a-covid-19-mrna-vaccine-technology-transfer-hub-to-scale-up -global-manufacturing (accessed 26 May 2022).
39. 'CARBIS BAY G7 SUMMIT COMMUNIQUÉ', The White House, https:// www.whitehouse.gov/briefing-room/statements-releases/2021/06/13/carbis-bay -g7-summit-communique/ (accessed 31 May 2022).
40. See: http:// www .millenniumpost .in/ sundaypost/ inland/ preventing -pitfalls -488694?infinitescroll=1 (accessed 17 August 2022).
41. See: https:// www .businesswire .com/ news/ home/ 20230117005286/ en/ Pfizer -Expands-%E2%80%98An-Accord-for-a-Healthier-World%E2%80%99-Product -Offering-to-Include-Full-Portfolio-for-Greater-Benefit-to-1.2-Billion-People-in-45 -Lower-Income-Countries (accessed 1 February 2023).
42. 'Feature: Chinese company wins acclaim for technology transfer endeavors to drive Ethiopia's fight against COVID-19', *People's Daily Online*, http://en .people.cn/n3/2022/0518/c90000-10098043.html (accessed 30 September 2022).
43. Gerald Chan, *China's maritime Silk Road: advancing global development?* (Cheltenham, UK, and Northampton, MA, USA: Edward Elgar Publishing, 2020), p. 4.
44. China's long history in Africa, *New African Magazine*, https://newafricanmagazine .com/ 10204/#:~:text=Historians%20and%20archaeologists%20are%20unsure ,point%20of%20Sino%2DAfrican%20relations (accessed 1 November 2022).
45. Liu Zhirong, 'What do Africans think of the Chinese', 2009, translated by David Cowhig, https://gaodawei.wordpress.com/2016/05/19/ (accessed 20 June 2022).
46. See: https://www.sahistory.org.za/ dated -event/ arrival -chinese -labourers -south -africa (accessed 10 August 2022).
47. See: http:// www .sais -cari .org/ data -chinese -workers -in -africa (accessed 18 August 2022). As of 2019, 182 745 Chinese nationals were working in Africa on various projects and in doing various businesses.
48. 'China in Africa: special report', *The Economist*, 28 May 2022, p. 3.

49. See: https:// www .globaltimes .cn/ page/ 202206/ 1269179 .shtml (accessed 7 December 2022).

50. Kaush Arha, 'The G7's $600 billion response to China's Belt and Road Initiative is here. This is how to make sure it succeeds', *New Atlanticist*, 8 November 2022.

51. 'Old wine in new bottles? China, the G7 and the new infrastructure geopolitics', ODI: Think change, https:// odi .org/ en/ insights/ old-wine-in-new-bottles-china -the-g7-and-the-new-infrastructure-geopolitics/ (accessed 14 December 2022).

52. For a good summary of China's recent assistance to Africa and the African Union, especially in dealing with the Covid-19 pandemic, see http://download .china.cn/en/pdf/en%E4%BB%8E%E5%85%B3%E9%94%AE%E8%AF%8D %E8%AF%BB%E6%87%82%E2%80%9C%E5%85%A8%E7%90%83%E5 %8F%91%E5%B1%95%E5%80%A1%E8%AE%AE%E2%80%9D%E7%A0 %94%E7%A9%B6%E6%8A%A5%E5%91%8A%20(1).pdf, p. 25 (accessed 16 September 2022).

53. Li Anshan, 'Chinese medical cooperation in Africa', Nordiska Afrikainstitutet, Uppsala, 2011.

54. See: https:// www .chinadaily .com .cn/ a/ 202209/ 09/ WS631b 3778a310fd 2b29e76f29.html (accessed 2 November 2022).

55. *China and Africa in the new era: A partnership of equals*, https://www.fmprc .gov .cn/ mfa _eng/ wjdt_665385/ 2649 _665393/ 202111/ t20211126 _10453904 .html (accessed 12 January 2023).

56. *China and Africa in the new era.*

57. His presentation at a Zoom conference on 'China's engagement in Africa's healthcare system' held at Georgetown University in Washington, DC, on 22 April 2022, https://www.youtube.com/watch?v=q3n_G5xHFIM (accessed 21 August 2022).

58. See: https://www.whitecase.com/insight-our-thinking/chinas-pivotal-role-supporting -post-covid-growth-africa (accessed 1 November 2022).

59. Components of these nine programmes can be found in Zhang Yiming, 'China–Africa cooperation enters a new stage and implements a new plan', 21 January 2022, http://na.china-embassy.gov.cn/eng/dsxx/hdjh/202201/t20220121 _10631816.htm (accessed 7 July 2022).

60. For the vision statement, see http://www.focac.org/eng/zywx_1/zywj/202201/ t20220124_10632442.htm (accessed 7 July 2022).

61. See: https://www.aljazeera.com/news/2021/11/29/chinas-xi-promises-1-billion -covid-19-vaccine-doses-to-africa (accessed 21 February 2023).

62. Zhang Yiming, 'China–Africa cooperation enters a new stage and implements a new plan', 21 January 2022.

63. See: https:// www .globaltimes .cn/ page/ 202301/ 1283618 .shtml (accessed 17 January 2023).

64. 'China-aided Africa CDC Headquarters main building marks structural comple- tion', *Xinhuanet*, 27 November 2021.

65. See: https:// moderndiplomacy .eu/ 2022/ 12/ 07/ china -signs -agreement -to -build -ecowas-headquarters/ (accessed 8 December 2022).

66. 'Vaccinating the world still needs coordination and cooperation that's in short supply', editorial board, *East Asia Forum*, 21 February 2022.

67. See: https:// www .cidrap .umn .edu/ news -perspective/ 2020/ 01/ china -releases -genetic-data-new-coronavirus-now-deadly (accessed 3 September 2022).

68. See: https://www.scmp.com/news/china/diplomacy/article/3174162/china-was -worlds-biggest-covid-19-vaccine-exporter-not-any (accessed 5 June 2022).

69. The statistics in this and the following paragraphs are sourced from Bridge Consulting, Beijing, https://bridgebeijing.com/our-publications/our-publications-1/china-covid-19-vaccines-tracker/ (accessed 21 February 2023).
70. Bridge Consulting stopped tracking on 28 December 2022.
71. Sourced from Bridge Consulting, Beijing.
72. Sourced from Bridge Consulting, Beijing.
73. See: https:// bridgebeijing .com/ blogposts/ fill -finish -and -beyond -how -chinese -vaccine-developers-are-exporting-their-ambitions-overseas/ (accessed 9 June 2022).
74. See: https://www.statista.com/statistics/421394/revenue-by-category-of-sinopharm/ (accessed 15 June 2022).
75. See: https://www.pharmaceutical-technology.com/news/pfizer-full-year-2021 -revenues/ (accessed 17 August 2022).
76. 'Vaccinating the world still needs coordination and cooperation that's in short supply'.
77. See: https://www.afdb.org/pt/news-and-events/press-releases/biovac-and-development -partners -collaborate -support -south -africas -vaccine -manufacturing -expansion -and -advance-long-term-health-security-across-africa-49641 (accessed 10 July 2022).
78. See: https://www.afdb.org/pt/news-and-events/press-releases/biovac-and-development -partners-collaborate-support-south-africas-vaccine-manufacturing-expansion-and -advance-long-term-health-security-across-africa-49641 (accessed 10 July 2022).
79. 'China, SA cooperation during Covid-19 a game changer?', *The Star*, South Africa, 6 April 2022.
80. See: https:// chinaglobalsouth .com/ analysis/ qa -is -china -really -delivering -for -senegal-in-the-fight-against-covid-19/ (accessed 10 July 2022).
81. See: https:// www .africanews .com/ 2021/ 06/ 07/ senegal -to -start -manufacturing -covid-19-vaccines/ (accessed 10 July 2022).
82. 'Morocco starts construction of COVID vaccine plant', *Aljazeera*, 28 January 2022; 'Morocco's Sothema to produce China's Sinopharm vaccine', *Reuters*, 6 July 2021.
83. Dubai was another staging point for China's air dispatch of vaccines and medical supplies to other parts of the world.
84. See: https://qz.com/africa/1834670/chinese-medical-aid-for-covid-19-in-africa -gets-mixed-support/ (accessed 10 July 2022).
85. See: https:// www .theafricareport .com/ 26750/ coronavirus -diplomacy -chinas -opportune-time-to-aid-africa/ (accessed 10 July 2022); https://www.alizila.com/ factsheet -jack -ma -foundation -alibaba -foundations -coronavirus -donations -and -efforts/ (accessed 11 November 2022).
86. 'Pandemic philanthropy: exploring Chinese donors' embrace of Covid-19 R&D funding', Bridge Consulting, Beijing, June 2020, pp. 8–9.
87. 'Pandemic philanthropy', pp. 8–9.
88. 'Philanthropy for sustainable development in China 2020', UNDP, Beijing, 2020, p. v.
89. Although China has a long traditional practice of filial piety to one's family and relatives and loyalty to one's hometown which might have provided a motivation for contemporary philanthropy.
90. See: https://www.alliancemagazine.org/blog/philanthropy-with-chinese-characteristics -through-the-lens-of-health/ (accessed 25 July 2022). According to the UNDP, the total number of foundations was 4932 in 2015, rising to 5760 in 2016, 6495 in

2017, and 7190 in 2018. 'Philanthropy for sustainable development in China 2020', p. 12.

91. See: https://www.pishu.cn/zxzx/xwdt/584004.shtml, quoted in 'Philanthropy cooperation: a bright spot in China–US relations', *The Diplomat*, 7 September 2022.

92. See: https://www.hurun.net/en-US/Info/Detail?num=LWAS8B997XUP (accessed 25 July 2022).

93. See: https://www.businessinsider.in/finance/news/list-of-top-20-richest-people-in-the-world/articleshow/74475220.cms (accessed 11 November 2022).

94. See: https://www.investopedia.com/articles/investing/012715/5-richest-people-world.asp (accessed 15 December 2022).

95. See: https://ideas.darden.virginia.edu/china-billionaire-list (accessed 2 October 2022).

96. 'China's super-rich see fortunes plunge as economy slows', *The Asahi Shimbun*, 8 November 2022.

97. See: https://inequality.org/great-divide/updates-billionaire-pandemic/ (accessed 24 November 2022).

98. 'Pandemic philanthropy', p. 13.

99. 'Pandemic philanthropy', p. 13.

100. 'An analysis of Chinese charitable trusts in 2020: pandemic-driven development', *China Development Brief*, 10 October 2020.

101. See: https:// www .prnewswire .com/ news -releases/ 2021 -sees -online -charity -donations-soar-to-10-billion-rmb-in-china-301551885.html (accessed 25 July 2022).

102. See https:// www .hkihss .hku .hk/ en/ events/ seminar -by -dr -jacqueline -lin -20220920/ (accessed 13 September 2022). Also, Gerald Chan, *China's digital Silk Road: setting standards, powering growth* (Cheltenham, UK, and Northampton, MA, USA: Edward Elgar Publishing, 2022), Chapter 5 on digital economy and the e-yuan, esp. pp. 69–72.

103. For some elaboration of 'common prosperity', see Chan, *China's digital Silk Road*, pp. 148–50 and 164. See also Bert Hofman, 'Common prosperity', in Frank N. Pieke and Bert Hofman (eds), *CPC futures: the new era of socialism with Chinese characteristics* (Singapore: NUS epress, 2022), pp. 113–20.

104. 'Why are China's billionaires suddenly feeling so generous?', *Aljazeera*, 16 July 2021.

105. See: https://www.worldometers.info/world-population/africa-population/ (accessed 1 May 2023).

106. See: https://www.avmi-africa.org/ (accessed 19 July 2022).

107. African Union and Africa CDC, 'Partnerships for African Vaccine Manufacturing (PAVM) Framework for Action', 2022 (Version 1), p. 2.

108. African Union and Africa CDC, p. 11.

109. See: https://www.reuters.com/business/healthcare-pharmaceuticals/africa-needs -make-own-vaccines-hurdles-are-high-experts-say-2021-12-07/ (accessed 27 July 2022).

110. African Union and Africa CDC, 'Partnerships', p. 8. UK Aid has a different take though: The African vaccine market could grow from US$1.3 billion today to about US$2.3–5.4 billion by 2030. See 'Vaccine manufacturing in Africa', DCVMN member briefing – presentation document, UK Aid, 17 March 2021, p. 12.

111. Michel Sidibé, 'Vaccine inequity: ensuring Africa is not left out', in Aloysius Uche Ordu, *Foresight Africa: top priorities for the continent in 2022* (Africa Growth Initiative at Brookings, 2022), p. 32.

112. Carl Manlan, 'This is the key to boosting economic growth in Africa', World Economic Forum, 22 May 2019.

113. With the financial support of the German Development Cooperation, the construction of Ghana's first vaccine manufacturing plant is scheduled to begin in July 2022. Full operation is expected by January 2024 as a 'fill-and-finish' site. 'Ghana: construction of Ghana's first vaccine manufacturing plant begins in July', *Ghanaian Times*, Accra, 11 April 2022.

114. African Union and Africa CDC, 'Partnerships', p. 81.

115. See: https://bhekisisa.org/article/2021-11-04-how-africa-plans-to-make-60-of-the-vaccines-needed-on-the-continent/ (accessed 15 June 2022).

116. 'Vaccine manufacturing in Africa', pp. 24, 32.

117. 'Vaccine manufacturing in Africa', pp. 24, 32.

118. See: https://english.ahram.org.eg/News/476668.aspx (accessed 1 May 2023).

119. 'Africa CDC warns COVID-19 vaccine production could cease', *The Lancet*, Vol. 399, 30 April 2022.

120. 'Africa CDC warns'.

121. See: https://www.bmj.com/company/newsroom/who-efforts-to-bring-vaccine-manufacturing -to -africa -is -being -undermined -by -pharma -reveals -the -bmj/ (accessed 27 July 2022).

122. 'WHO pushes new COVID vaccine technologies', *China Daily*, 22 July 2022, https://www.chinadaily.com.cn/a/202203/01/WS621d7d0ba310cdd39bc897c1.html (accessed 11 December 2023).

123. 'Aspen's Covid-19 flop bodes ill for Africa vaccine making drive', Bloomberg, 18 May 2022.

124. 'Covid in Africa: Why the continent's only vaccine plant is struggling', BBC, 6 May 2022.

125. See: https://www.nytimes.com/2022/12/08/health/covid-vaccines-covax-gavi.html (accessed 14 December 2022).

126. *New York Times*, quoted in 'Is big pharma profiteering from the pandemic?', The University of Auckland (accessed 3 March 2023).

127. 'S. Africa's Aspen and India's Serum Institute sign vaccines deal for Africa', *Reuters*, 1 September 2022.

128. Wang Xiaoyi, 'China, not COVAX, led vaccine exports to the world's middle income countries in 2021', 10 February 2022, https://healthpolicy-watch.news/china-covax-led-vaccine-exports-lmic-2021/ (accessed 1 August 2022).

129. Wang, 2022.

130. Gerald Chan, Pak K. Lee, and Chan Lai-Ha, *China engages global governance: a new world order in the making?* (London and New York: Routledge, 2012), pp. 114–17.

131. See: https://www.ncbi.nlm.nih.gov/pmc/articles/PMC7153452/ (accessed 8 September 2022).

132. Tang Zhimin and Orrasa Rattana-amornpirom, 'The BRI in the new normal of COVID-19: the case of Thailand', in Joseph Chinyong Liow, Liu Hong and Gong Xue (eds), *Research handbook on the Belt and Road Initiative* (Cheltenham, UK, and Northampton, MA, USA, 2022), pp. 209–10.

133. See: https://www.statista.com/chart/21372/assessed-contributions-to-the-world-health-organization/ (accessed 30 December 2022).

134. See: https://www.statista.com/chart/21372/assessed-contributions-to-the-world -health-organization/ (accessed 30 December 2022).

135. See: https://www.cnbc.com/2021/02/17/us-will-pay-who-more-than-200-million -in-membership-fees-withheld-by-trump.html (accessed 4 September 2022).

136. See: https://www.who.int/about/funding (accessed 19 August 2022).

137. See: http://download.china.cn/en/pdf/en%E4%BB%8E%E5%85%B3%E9%94 %AE%E8%AF%8D%E8%AF%BB%E6%87%82%E2%80%9C%E5%85%A8 %E7%90%83%E5%8F%91%E5%B1%95%E5%80%A1%E8%AE%AE%E2 %80%9D%E7%A0%94%E7%A9%B6%E6%8A%A5%E5%91%8A%20(1) .pdf, p. 23 (accessed 16 September 2022).

138. See: https://www.who.int/director-general/who-headquarters-leadership-team (accessed 4 September 2022).

139. See: https://www.who.int/china/health-topics/health-financing (accessed 4 September 2022).

140. See: http://english.www.gov.cn/statecouncil/ministries/202101/28/content_WS6012 b1f1c6d0f72576944b2d.html (accessed 4 September 2022).

141. 'Development of China's public health as an essential element of human rights', White Paper, Information Office, State Council, PRC, September 2017.

142. See: https://www.who.int/health-topics/international-health-regulations#tab=tab _1 (accessed 16 May 2022).

143. A monkeypox virus is usually endemic in Central and West Africa. Since mid-May 2022, monkeypox cases have been increasingly reported in non-endemic countries, starting from Europe, North America, and Australia. Information from the Department of Health, Hong Kong SAR, displayed at the Hong Kong International Airport, as of 19 October 2022.

144. See: https://www.mfa.gov.cn/ce/cesg/eng/whjyykj/kjjl/t1888893.htm (accessed 27 July 2022).

145. See: https://www.fmprc.gov.cn/mfa_eng/wjdt_665385/2649_665393/202106/ t20210624_9170568.html (accessed 18 August 2022).

146. See: https://www.fmprc.gov.cn/mfa_eng/xwfw_665399/s2510_665401/2535 _665405/202108/t20210802_9170834.html (accessed 18 August 2022).

147. For a description of the origins and development of LOGINK, see Chan, *China's digital Silk Road*, pp. 20–23.

148. See: https://www.ich.org/ (accessed 30 December 2022).

149. NMPA holds symposium on process and prospects of ICH in China (accessed 30 December 2022).

150. See: https://www.business-standard.com/article/international/xi-jinping-announces -additional -1 -billion -for -global -development -fund -122062401047 _1 .html (accessed 19 September 2022).

151. In general, what Africa needs in terms of development, according to a Chinese expert He Wenping, are three things: infrastructure building; training and human resources; and investments. https://www.guancha.cn/HeWenPing/2023_01_16 _676060_1.shtml (accessed 18 January 2023).

6.   Patient rights vs patent rights

'It is easier for a camel to go through the eye of a needle than for a rich man to enter the kingdom of God', so says Jesus in the New Testament. His admonition reveals the predicament faced by the rich when they are confronted with demands to share their vaccines with those who are much less fortunate than they are in the fight against Covid-19.

The statistics make grim reading. As of 25 April 2022, 11.54 billion doses of Covid-19 vaccines had been administered globally. The majority of them went to the rich: 80 per cent of the people in high-income and upper-middle-income countries had received their first dose, and 60 per cent in lower-middle-income countries had received their first jab, but only 15 per cent in low-income countries had done so.[1] The Covid death toll in low-income countries was about four times that of the rich ones.[2] Facing such a situation, a challenge for all of us is that new variants of the virus would have ample opportunities to mutate and so continue to play havoc around the world with little or no respect for social-economic status or territorial boundaries. The WHO estimated that, as of October 2022, over 300 Covid variants might push to form a new wave of infections in some countries around the world.[3]

Clearly, the rich are well protected because of their wealth and their near monopoly of patent rights over life-saving drugs, while the poor have been suffering and will likely continue to suffer disproportionally from the lack of access to those drugs. This is not a situation arising from the outbreak of Covid-19 only, it has been a long-standing problem in the history of the modern world. This chapter asks: What actually are the patient rights in public health? Are they health rights? Or are they human rights? On the other hand, what are patent rights? Are these two sets of rights at odds with each other? Need they be? Can they be made compatible with each other? To what extent can that be done? How has China – a rising power in drug manufacturing and a major vaccine exporter – positioned itself in this dichotomy?

ARE HEALTH RIGHTS HUMAN RIGHTS?

The right to health is probably as old as human rights itself, but the linkage between the two has only been made more explicit since the onset of industrialisation and the Enlightenment in modern Europe. Legal-authoritative references to health rights in contemporary times can be found in the Universal

Declaration of Human Rights (1948) and in such international treaties as the International Covenant on Economics, Social, and Cultural Rights (1966) and the International Covenant on Civil and Political Rights (1966). Together, these three legal documents make up the International Bill of Rights. The International Covenant on Economics, Social, and Cultural Rights stipulates that everyone has a right to 'the enjoyment of the highest attainable standard of physical and mental health' (Article 12.1). This stipulation seems clear enough, but what may not be so clear is the meaning of the word *highest* – how high is high and how absolute or measurable is the standard used to gauge the degree of highness?

Major international bodies like the WHO also champion the right to health. The Constitution of the WHO, entered into force in 1948, says that 'The enjoyment of the highest attainable standard of health is one of the fundamental rights of every human being without distinction of race, religion, political belief, economic or social condition'.[4] To the WHO, 'the right to health for all people means that everyone should have access to the health services they need, when and where they need them'.[5] As such, health rights are treated as universal rights.

How have health rights come into conflict with patent rights? To answer this question, perhaps a good starting point would be the year of 1994 when the WTO formulated the Agreement on Trade and Related Aspects of Intellectual Property Rights (TRIPS). This agreement is the latest consolidation of patents and intellectual property (IP) as rights. It works to standardise worldwide IP laws, including laws that deal with pharmaceutical products, in addition to others such as computer software, entertainment, and agribusiness – industries that topped the agenda of trade disputes at the time. It sets out the terms to protect the rights of property owners and patent holders. These owners and holders are mostly wealthy people living and working in the West enjoying the *highest* standard of living. In the case of pharmaceutical products, patent holders are mostly big drug companies and their major shareholders. Most countries in the developing world have been forced to accept the TRIPS arrangement under immense pressure exerted by rich countries, including the use of trade threats.

India seems to be a curious exception to the rule among developing countries. This exception has important implications for the development of more affordable generic drugs for the global poor as well as for many people among the global rich. Before the inception of TRIPS, India did not recognise the patent coverage of pharmaceutical products under its own Patents Act of 1970 and its subsequent amendments.[6] Since its independence from Great Britain in 1947, India has been fiercely defending its self-reliance on vaccines and therapeutics. The Serum Institute, now the world's biggest vaccine manufacturer, was founded in 1966 in the city of Pune, in western India near Mumbai.

Coupled with the country's investment restrictions in the 1970s and 1980s,[7] this fierce resistance to British control helped to usher in the development of a strong generic drug industry in the newly independent country.[8] It was only in 1994 that India and the WTO signed an agreement to require the country to institute, by 1 January 2005, patents on pharmaceutical products rather than on the process of making them.[9] India and many other developing countries were pressured or persuaded by rich countries to accept the TRIPS Agreement in exchange for WHO membership (the WHO replaced GATT, the General Agreement on Tariffs and Trade, in 1995) with incipient promises of hefty economic benefits to be had from free trade.[10]

What is the role of patents in relation to drugs? Patents play a huge role. They allow holders to exercise strict control over the production, sales, distribution, and pricing of drugs. During a patent life (ranging usually from 15 to 20 years), no one is legally allowed to produce, buy, or sell patented products without obtaining a licence from the patent holder. This inherently creates a monopoly, a situation which faces little challenge or competition from drug manufacturers in the Global South, although they may be in a position to produce many similar drugs at a much lower cost and sell them at a much lower price, which would benefit the poor. The temptation by patent holders to hike prices to maximise profits reduces the affordability and accessibility of life-saving drugs for the poor. Such an outcome challenges the obligations of states to provide adequate healthcare for their citizens. In a wider sense, the rights to health include not only the rights to have fair and easy access to medical treatments, but also 'access to safe drinking water and sanitation, nutritious foods, adequate housing, education and safe working conditions',[11] all of which play a part in the attainment of good health. So poverty is the main culprit of poor health outcomes.

Patent rights are generally regarded as private property rights, although some have argued that they are also human rights. Those who argue in defence of the status quo of monopoly to guarantee the fruits of invention and innovation in terms of monetary returns for initial investments in R&D appeal to the human right to 'the protection of the moral and material interests resulting from any scientific, literary or artistic production of which he [or she] is the author'. This is stipulated in the Universal Declaration of Human Rights (Article 27) and in the International Covenant on Economic, Social, and Cultural Rights (Article 15.1(c)).[12] So, in theory and in rare circumstances, a case can be made in which *one set of human rights could be used against another set of human rights* due to different preferences and different interpretations of what constitutes human rights and which component part of human rights is regarded as more important than the other(s).

Patent rights are designed to protect the interests derived from the IP of the inventors, and hence to protect the materially rich class that possesses those rights. Drug manufacturers are particularly keen to protect their patent rights and IP in the expectation of making quick, handsome profits from their investments – the very essence of capitalism (Chapter 3) and the nature of human greed, generally assumed and understood. Where do patent rights come from in the first place?

PATENT RIGHTS: ORIGINS AND DEVELOPMENT

Patents are essentially the ways and means to protect and promote the material interests of the inventor.[13] States grant them as exclusive rights to an inventor to exploit their invention. As such, they form a kind of reward or inducement that the state gives the inventor for their contribution to the solution of a problem in technology or industry. The inventor can decide to disclose and publicise their invention to society in exchange for the state's assurance that no one thereafter will be able to copy it without their consent for a certain period of time. Patents therefore perform a dual function: as an inducement to invent on the one hand; and as an essential factor of scientific and technological progress on the other. Pushed to their respective extremes, these two functions are at odds with each other. It can be argued, for example, that being *overly* protective of those rights could have the *undesirable* effect of narrowing the window of opportunities for newcomers to make inventions based on the latest innovation available, leading then to the stifling of competition and the slowing down of overall scientific progress.

Theoretically speaking, we can assume that all states want to protect the interests of inventors. In practice, this assumption can be challenged. In general, those states which are rich in innovation and inventions stand to benefit 'disproportionally' more if there are stringent rules to protect, not only within their own jurisdiction, but more importantly in the jurisdictions of other countries as well. However, those states which are less innovative would lose out because they have to pay large sums of money to acquire copyrights when they buy those heavily protected products, like life-saving drugs. In other words, rich developed countries earn a lot of income while poor developing countries pay a lot of money when they buy well-protected goods and services. This is the reason why poor countries are reluctant to sign up to TRIPS. But they have little choice, as rich and powerful states exert a lot of political and economic pressure on them. The TRIPS Agreement is often seen as a successful conclusion of lengthy trade talks and negotiations among members of the WTO in the process of multilateral cooperation and globalisation, which is not entirely without foundation, but, in many respects, it can also be seen as a triumph of the rich over the poor, especially when the poor are in a weak and vulnerable position.

The ideas of individualism, individual rights (of an inventor), and scientific progress are very much the ideational fruits of (Western) modernisation. Although the concept of patents came out of European commercial experiences in the 15th century or earlier, it was the Industrial Revolution of the 18th century that sped up manufacturing processes and started the modern era of patenting. The US Congress passed its Patent Act in 1790. A year later, France passed the French Law that treated inventors' rights as sacred and inviolable.

The issue of patent rights of pharmaceutical products is particularly controversial, for three reasons: first, these products relate to important issues of human health, sometimes of a life-and-death nature. Second, many resources are being ploughed into the process of inventing and the testing of new drugs, so there is an extra demand for the protection of their investments and patents. And third, drugs are relatively easy to be replicated and mass produced once their chemical formula is known.

To recap, arguments have focused on two main opposing stands: first, the primacy of the rights of patent holders and, second, the primacy of the rights of patients to life and well-being. The rights of patents hold that R&D of drugs takes up a lot of time and resources, and therefore holders of patents should have the rights to protect their IP and to reap the rewards of their investments. To take away their rights would detract entrepreneurs, investors, and inventors from developing new drugs to tackle future diseases. This would then retard human progress.

The counterargument that favours the rights of patients stresses the importance of saving lives, pointing out that the right to health and, hence, the right to access affordable drugs are paramount, overriding the rights to monetary gains and profits. Many nuanced arguments have also been made over time based on various economic and legal reasons. The issue is complex. Arguments and opinions are very much anchored in different understandings of human values. There seems to be little or no consensus as to the best way forward to resolve this dilemma.

When countries reach a certain advanced stage of industrial development, they tend to pass or strengthen domestic patent laws to protect their IP. In contemporary times, examples include France in 1960, Germany in 1968, Japan in 1976, Switzerland in 1977, and Italy in 1978.[14] Nearly all the countries in the West and the North have signed up to protect patent rights from the 1970s to the 1990s. China is a latecomer to this patent community, joining the WTO and the TRIPS Agreement only in 2001 after lengthy discussions and negotiations with developed countries, especially the US, to set the terms and conditions of China's entry into the world body.

Patent rights have become the rights for the rich and powerful to protect their property. To the poor, however, these rights have become an instrument of capitalist exploitation, a mechanism of monopolistic control. Arguments raging in the Uruguay Round of multilateral trade negotiations from 1986 to 1994 ended with the creation of the WTO in 1995 and the adoption of the TRIPS Agreement. Apart from a few very poor countries in the world,[15] nearly all countries have now adopted domestic legislation to comply with TRIPS, although different countries have followed different timetables to do so, due to their different stages of development and, hence, different capacities to comply. In addition, rich countries in the world, in particular the US, have moved further ahead to protect their patent rights beyond TRIPS by forging bilateral trade agreements and regional trade agreements to consolidate and enhance their (privileged) positions, a phenomenon that analysts in the field call 'TRIPS-Plus' provisions. The effects of these provisions are yet to be fully felt because they are relatively new (yet to be tested) and because different provisions are being applied to different countries, and they have different timings for implementation.[16]

Despite different views on the pros and cons of patents and divergent policies to legislate the protection of IP among countries, it was agreed that by 2005 patents for pharmaceutical products would be adopted worldwide. Those countries that did not grant them but were members of the WTO would then be exposed to the dispute settlement procedures within the world trading body. They would be subject to possible corresponding economic reprisals.[17] Apart from wielding power – formal or informal – through the WTO, rich countries can, of course, resort to using unilateral action to punish poor countries for non-compliance, for example, what the US has done in its trade (war) with China, accusing China of stealing IP, among numerous other charges (see Chapter 7 for more).

PATENT RIGHTS VS PATIENT RIGHTS

Are patent rights and patient rights diametrically opposed to each other? Can they coexist in some way? Do countries have to choose between them?

This paradox arose probably as early as the development of medicinal drugs themselves. The awareness of the right to gain access to life-saving drugs to fight pandemics comes about when the supply of these drugs has become short, resulting in a quick and broad spread of diseases, especially in communities where members can ill afford to buy those drugs, for financial or other social-cultural reasons.

To alleviate the conflict between patent rights and patient rights, two major options have been devised. They are designated as 'flexibilities'[18] in the TRIPS system: compulsory licensing and patent waiver.[19] Apart from these two approaches, many other measures are used by stakeholders to deal with the conflict. They include, among others, parallel imports, patent pools, technology transfer, and, in the case of Covid-19, COVAX – a programme to collect the contributions made by multiple donors and organised by international health organisations. A parallel option is a non-counterfeit product imported from another country without the permission of the IP owner.[20] A patent pool, on the other hand, is 'an agreement between two or more patent owners to license one or more of their patents to one another or to third parties'.[21] What then are compulsory licensing and patent waiver, the two major flexibilities for poor countries to adopt to relieve their pain and to avoid the scourge of deadly diseases?

Compulsory Licensing

A compulsory licence is a permission granted by a state authority allowing a third party to use a patented invention without the consent of the patent holder.[22] It is regarded as a non-voluntary agreement between a voluntary buyer and a non-voluntary seller, imposed and enforced by a state for public health benefits.[23] Such agreements between parties often involve different states, that is, a buyer from one state and a seller from another, and so these agreements can take many forms due to the complexities arising from cross-border and cross-jurisdictional arrangements. Such agreements have been made possible as the state is allowed to invoke authority provided for by the TRIPS Agreement – to authorise a third party to import and distribute drugs for 'public non-commercial use' or for 'government use' or national emergency, without seeking the approval of the relevant patent holders. The state, however, has to pay the rights holder an adequate amount of remuneration as a compensation, in line with the guidelines laid down by the WHO for calculating such remunerations. In practice, the state and the patent holder would have to enter into agreed arrangements to do so. The process is often cumbersome and there are certain ramifications and consequences of taking a particular course of action. Because of the complex process involved and because life is often at stake in a crisis situation in which a quick decision is called for, some states would prefer or demand the outright waiving of patent rights so that the necessary pharmaceutical products can be obtained speedily at an affordable price.

Intellectual Property Waiver

IP waiver is an option preferred by most developing countries as a way to overcome the harsh restrictions set by compulsory licensing. Such harsh restrictions include a product-by-product identification of medical materials, the long time required to identify the relevant patents, the burdensome process of going through various government departments, the constraints put on the marketing of the medical products concerned, the length of the waiver period, and the difficulties involved in settling on the amount of renumeration for rights owners.[24] The list goes on and on.

IP waiver sounds reasonable and fair to the world's poor but not so to the rich in an apparently very tight negative-sum game. To negotiate or give away the rights of patent holders means ultimately to diminish their opportunity to make significant profits, an opportunity that has grown out of the development of capitalism in the West buttressed by a *robust and powerful* legal system, international as well as domestic. (See Jesus's parabolic saying at the beginning of this chapter!) It has been reported that Pfizer, BioNTech, and Moderna, the three big Covid vaccine manufacturers in the world, would together make pre-tax profits of US$34 billion in 2021, which works out to be over $1000 a second, or $65 000 a minute, or $93.5 million a day.[25] The history of patents and the controversies surrounding the case of Covid-19 have amply demonstrated the difficulties involved in securing IP waivers on drugs.

Between Waiving and Licensing: The Covid Case

A recent case concerning Covid vaccines illustrates well the practical difficulties and complexities involved in the patent-versus-patient conflict. In October 2020 the Indian and South African governments put forward a joint proposal to the WTO to waive IP protection in order to scale up the production of medical supplies such as vaccines, medicines, and test kits for the duration of the Covid-19 pandemic.[26] This proposal was widely supported by developing countries,[27] with 65 members of the WTO co-sponsoring it and 110 countries backing it.[28] However, it was strongly opposed by the EU, Switzerland, and the UK, where some of the world's biggest pharmaceutical companies reside or operate. The US, originally siding with other Western countries, turned around to support the proposal in May 2021, with a view to boost the production and distribution of Covid vaccines around the world.[29]

Various reasons have been put forward to argue for or against an IP waiver. Those who argue for an IP waiver stress, in the main, the importance of producing enough accessible medical supplies fast enough to save as many lives as possible. Those who argue against warn that waiving patents would jeopardise incentives to invent new vaccines to tackle future pandemics. Specifically, those WTO members who argue against an IP waiver have pointed out that[30]:

- An IP waiver will lower the quality of Covid medical products;
- There is no evidence that IP is a barrier to vaccine access; and
- The implementation of an IP waiver would affect innovation.

Negotiations, debates, and mutual recriminations have been raging fiercely over complex legal, economic, and political issues. The WTO, especially under its new Director-General Ngozi Okonjo-Iweala, a former Nigerian minister of finance who assumed her headship in March 2021, was keen to find a way out to resolve the disputes over TRIPS waiver among member states.

In March 2022 the US, the EU, India, and South Africa reached a compromise, mediated by the WTO secretariat in Geneva. A document setting out the terms was said to have leaked to the media. Many academics and social activists were quick to point out the shortcomings of the compromise. These include[31]:

1. The text applies only to patents on vaccines, and only for Covid-19, not other medicines, diagnostics, and therapeutics.
2. Eligibility is limited to WTO developing countries that exported less than 10 per cent of the world's vaccines in 2021. This means that China would be automatically excluded, as its share of the global exports of Covid-19 vaccines is about 34 per cent,[32] if not more. Brazil too would be excluded as it has recently surrendered its developing country status in exchange for US support to enter the OECD.[33]
3. Various conditions and complications that hinder the scaling up of vaccine production, the cumbersome application for licences, the reluctance to transfer technology,[34] and the difficulties in reaching agreements on compensations and renumerations.

The compromised text was put to WTO members for deliberation. A consensus of all 164 members was needed for it to be adopted – a basic principle of the trade body to make a major decision. Many critics of the compromise, including NGOs such as MSF (Medecins sans Frontieres or Doctors without Borders), recommended a rejection because of the harsh terms and conditions.[35] Eventually, at a ministerial meeting on 17 June 2022,[36] the WTO members reached an agreement on an IP waiver. As a result, it removes a ban on exporting vaccines procured under a compulsory licence. Poor countries can now theoretically commence to make vaccines without seeking patent approval from patent holders, subject to payment of mutually agreed royalties. It was, however, regarded by some analysts as a half-baked agreement. No one seems to be entirely happy with the outcome because of its limitations: it applies only to Covid-19 vaccines within a five-year period; and diagnostics and therapeutics are to be discussed in six months' time. China is barred from a waiver, a key US demand aimed at preventing China from 'stealing mRNA technology'.

mRNA stands for messenger ribonucleic acid, a relatively new technology that stimulates an immune response and is considered the most effective method of treatment. China is developing its own mRNA vaccines.[37] While still at the stage of clinical trials, Chinese mRNA vaccines were approved for emergency use by Indonesia in September 2022, the first country to do so.[38] In February 2023 Reuters reported that CanSino, a Chinese pharma company, was confident that its mRNA Covid vaccine, still under active trial, would be as effective as those already being widely used in the world.[39] In March 2023, BBC reported that China approved its first homemade mRNA Covid vaccine.[40] In the meantime, the US leads in the R&D of mRNA. It has 688 patent families relating to mRNA, while China has 336 and Germany 233. Together these three countries account for 72 per cent of the global total mRNA patents.[41]

CHINESE VIEWS ON HEALTH RIGHTS

The idea of rights based on individuals as units in society originated in Western thought and practice through centuries of political, economic, cultural, and scientific developments: from the Great Charter and the Industrial Revolution to the Enlightenment, the French Revolution, and the American Revolution – a 600-year history of progression. Such a trend of thought and practice is largely alien to the vast majority of the Chinese and many other peoples in the developing world, apart from a relatively small group of cosmopolitan-minded, Western-educated, and well-informed elites. In this context, the health policy of China today has inevitably inherited the legacies of traditional Chinese thought and practice, and it is now also subject to the influence of the political ideology of the PRC. Its health policy is very much designed to provide medical services to the general public in a mass-campaign style, for demographic and historical reasons – focusing relatively more on basic services than specific pathological ones, more on collective treatment than individual care, in comparison with the West. The massive lockdowns and the zero-Covid policy could perhaps be partly seen in this light. (The long-term effects of ditching the zero-Covid policy in December 2022 and the lifting of travel bans – both domestic and international – since January 2023 are yet to be fully felt. At least in February, the government declared a 'decisive victory' over Covid.[42] And GDP growth in the first quarter of 2023 was up 4.5 per cent over the same period a year earlier,[43] a higher growth rate than many forecasts predicted. Most forecasts for China's economic growth for 2023 ranged from 5.2 per cent to 5.7 per cent.[44]) The prevention of diseases remains a priority, with the help of both TCM and Western medicine.[45] China's opening to the outside world, including to the UN family, specifically the WHO and the WTO, has pushed the country to align more than ever before with the rules and regulations of global health development shaped in large part by Western ideas and practices.

China regards health rights as human rights, but more in terms of development rights and economic rights than civil and political rights. Of the three generations of human rights, China places greater importance on development rights, followed by economic, social, and cultural rights, and only then by civil and political rights. China prefers this priority, as it aspires to become, first and foremost, a strong and rich nation powered by development and modernisation. Indeed, it has achieved success in the area of growth and development, especially in the past 40 years or so as a result of reform and opening up. The development of its civil and political rights, in contrast, though making some progress, is relatively weak, certainly so when measured using Western standards and expectations. The country, however, has beaten a new, effective path of development, to the admiration of many developing countries. They have looked towards China as a model for emulation. I have proposed a concept called geo-developmentalism as a framework for analysing China's BRI,[46] including its HSR. It is a concept that tries to capture China's efforts to develop trade through building infrastructure connections. China signed the International Covenant on Economic, Social, and Cultural Rights in 1997 and ratified it in 2001. It also signed the International Covenant on Civil and Political Rights in 1998 but has yet to ratify it as of August 2023.[47]

China's white paper on public health (2017) states that 'the right to health is a basic human right … Everyone is entitled to the highest standard of health, equally available and accessible'.[48] In 2019 the National People's Congress (China's parliament) passed the *Basic Healthcare and Health Promotion Law*. This piece of legislation is the most important one so far, in the sense that it has summed up China's health policy and given it a legal status. It formally overhauls the health laws and codifies various ambitious health reform programmes in the past decade, especially the Healthy China 2030 initiative. The Law declares that both 'State and society' shall 'respect and protect citizens' right to health'. It aims to promote knowledge about health, optimise the delivery of healthcare services, and lift the level of health of the people in a 'complete cycle of life' (from cradle to grave).[49] To a Chinese analyst, the emphasis on the right to health is broadly in line with international trends and the UN SDGs.[50]

China's stance on health rights as human rights appears clear in theory. In practice, however, the country does not seem to have been very active in translating its views on health rights into human rights in action and following them through, either alone or in partnership with other developing countries. For instance, China has not been very vocal or active in contributing to the process of IP waiver negotiations at the WHO, discussed above. Rather, it has chosen to work with other countries on a bilateral basis, or through the Belt and Road partnership or South–South cooperation like the BRICS or various regional forums with countries in Asia, Africa, the Middle East, and Latin America. The closest policy relating to an IP waiver as far as Covid-19 is concerned is the country's public announcement made by President Xi Jinping calling on the treating of Covid-19 vaccines as global public goods.

CHINESE VIEWS ON PATENT RIGHTS[51]

As China makes great advances in industrialisation, the protection and promotion of patent rights have assumed increasing attention, for its own interests and potentially for the interests of others as well. The country is, however, late coming to the highly competitive game of registering patents, royalties, and IP. Developed countries have built up a clear lead in this race: the US and Japan began filing their patents as early as the 1880s, South Korea started to file its own in the 1960s, and the European Patent Office did in the 1970s. (Of course, individual western European countries started much earlier.) China only started to do so in the 1980s, subsequent to its reform and opening up.[52] Since its entry into the WTO in 2001, Chinese patent applications have risen sharply, a trend that has continued up to this day.[53] Within a short period of time, China has registered a surge in patents granted by the World Intellectual Property Organization (WIPO): from 4919 in 2010 to 25 034 in 2017, narrowing the gap of foreign patent counts between itself and a number of OECD countries[54] (Table 6.1). Many Chinese patents are regarded by market analysts as of low quality. However, China has plans to improve the quality of its patents in future, aiming to nearly double its high-value invention patents from 6.3 pieces per 10 000 people in 2020 to 12 pieces by 2025.[55] These include inventions in strategic emerging industries and patent families – a collection of documents for the same invention – granted by foreign patent offices. Also, China plans to optimise its subsidies and performance evaluation system, incubate patent-intensive industries, and grant universities and state-owned enterprises greater autonomy and ownership in managing their IP.[56]

According to WIPO, in 2018 China received 46.4 per cent of all patent applications filed worldwide.[57] However, in terms of filing patents abroad (that is, excluding resident or domestic filings), the US led in the field, followed by Japan, Germany, South Korea, and then China.[58] The ranking changed quickly in 2019 when, for the first time, China surpassed the US to become the top filer of international patent applications.[59] (However, in terms of medicinal drugs, the top patent holders were Switzerland, the UK, and the US, as of 2019.[60]) If we add to the total mix by including trademarks and industrial designs in addition to patents, China would be clearly in the lead to become an IP powerhouse (Table 6.2). (A patent protects new, useful, and ingenious inventions. A trademark is a combination of letters, words, sounds, or designs that distinguishes one business's goods or services from those of others. And an industrial design registration provides protection for the original visual features of a product.[61])

Why and how has China moved so fast in the patent race? The country's recent development in the area of IP protection offers some clue. Patent law in contemporary China began with the promulgation of the Patent Law of the

Table 6.1 *Top three applicants of patents, trademarks, and industrial designs by origin, 2018–19*

	2018	2019
Patents		
Applications worldwide	3 325 400	3 224 200*
China	1 542 002	1 400 661
US	586 141	621 453
Japan	313 567	307 969
Trademarks		
Applications worldwide	14 314 000	15 153 700
China	7 365 352	7 833 081
US	640 100	672 681
Japan	512 106	546 244
Industrial designs		
Applications worldwide	1 343 800	1 360 990
China	708 799	711 617
EU office	108 553	113 319
South Korea	68 310	69 360

Notes: * Total granted worldwide: 1.5 million.
Patents in force worldwide as of 2019: 15 million, of which the US had 3.1 million, China 2.7 million, and Japan 2 million.
Source: World IP indicators 2020 (Geneva: WIPO, 2020), pp. 7, 19.

Table 6.2 *Top ten IP filings (resident and abroad) by origin, 2019*

Origin	Patents	Marks	Designs
China	1	1	1
US	2	2	4
Germany	5	4	2
Japan	3	3	8
South Korea	4	10	3
France	6	6	6
UK	7	7	9
Italy	11	13	5
India	10	8	13
Switzerland	8	14	10

Source: World IP indicators 2020 (Geneva: WIPO, 2020), p. 8.

Table 6.3   *Development of China's patent law with reference to drugs, 1984–2021*

Year	Legislation	Major issues relating to patents
1984	Patent Law	To stipulate the compulsory licensing system
1992	Patent Law (first amendment)	To expand to cover drugs
2000	Patent Law (second amendment)	To meet TRIPS Agreement requirements
2005	Measures for Compulsory Licence on Patent Implementation Concerning Public Health Problems	'Infectious diseases' to include SARS (outbreak in 2002), AIDS, tuberculosis, malaria, etc.
2008	Patent Law (third amendment)	A special chapter on compulsory licensing system
2010	Implementing Regulations of the Patent Law	Chapter 5 on the compulsory licensing of patent implementation
2012	Measures on Compulsory Licensing of Patent	To improve the system
2018	Opinions on Reforming and Improving Policies on the Supply Assurance and Use of Generic Drugs	To cover 'national emergency', 'shortage of drugs' and 'serious and critical diseases' such as cancer, cardiovascular diseases, etc.
2020	Patent Law (fourth amendment)	To incentivise rights owners; enhance design patents; provide anti-monopoly provisions
2021	Measures for the Implementation of the Early Resolution Mechanism of Drug Patent Disputes (trial)	Together with 'Judicial Interpretation on Patent Linkage and Administrative Adjudication Rules' and the amended Patent Law, they form the legal framework of China's patent linkage system

Source: Cao Zhang et al., 'The legislative approach and system improvement of China's compulsory licensing for drug patents', *Drug Design, Development and Therapy*, Dovepress, No. 15 (2021), pp. 3719–20. Updated with internet materials, 13 May 2022.

People's Republic of China in 1984. In the following year, the country acceded to the Paris Convention for the Protection of Industrial Property, followed by the Patent Cooperation Treaty in 1994. The Paris Convention, signed in 1883, was one of the first IP treaties. The Patent Cooperation Treaty, on the other hand, is an international patent law treaty. Concluded in 1970 in Washington, DC, and deposited with WIPO, it provides a unified procedure for filing patent applications to protect inventions in each of its contracting states. When China joined the WTO in 2001, it became a member of the TRIPS Agreement, which aims to protect trade-related IP. It has amended its Patent Law four times: in 1992, 2000, 2008, and 2020.[62] Table 6.3 summarises the legal development of China's compulsory licensing for drug patents, an important aspect of China's overall patent development relevant to this study.

China's patent linkage system, effective 1 June 2021, serves three main purposes[63]:

1. To protect the legitimate rights and interests of drug patentees;
2. To ensure the early settlement of patent disputes before generic drugs are listed; and
3. To reduce the risk of patent infringement after generic drugs are listed.

The development of China's patent system has been driven by external pressure, mainly from the US, and by China's own effort to fulfil its obligations as a new member of the WTO. Very quickly China has come to realise the importance of protecting its own copyrights and patent rights, so the country has taken steps to institute its legal system and to comply with international law. Over the past four decades or so, China has been quietly building up its patent system. It has learned from the international legal and regulatory framework to build its IP protocol, especially borrowing ideas from the German model. Through its BRI, it has also acquired experiences and knowledge of the patent systems from partner countries. So active and fast has China been involving itself in the development of the international patent regime that it is seen to be on the cusp of becoming the new IP superpower.[64]

However, China has yet to issue any compulsory licence for drug patents, although some developing countries have already been issuing such licences in relatively large numbers since the turn of the century. It has been reported that, since 2001, compulsory licensing of medicines has been used 34 times in 24 countries.[65] One plausible explanation for the Chinese reluctance in issuing such licensing relates to the lack of clear procedural provisions in the licensing law.[66] Another plausible explanation relates to the overly strict regulations on the scope of the object of compulsory licensing and on the qualification of applicants.[67] A third possibility is the low level of profits that can be generated by producing generic drugs in this way.[68] Nevertheless, the regularisation of its patent system has started to help the country to nurture the growth of its drug industry and enhance the export potentials of its pharmaceuticals as well as medical devices.

CONCLUSION

The rapid growth of China's pharmaceutical industry and the active promotion of its patent rights beg a couple of tricky questions: first, whether or not the Chinese government would take decisive steps to curb the growing wealth of Chinese investors in some specific health sectors to achieve greater economic equality and social stability in the country. The government has done this before with the hi-tech sector, especially in dealing with some big social media companies, using the idea of 'common prosperity' as a rationale to achieve social-economic goals. Second, whether or not it will share the wealth generated from its pharmaceutical industry with other developing countries. In the case of Covid-19, President Xi Jinping has pledged that the country would provide Covid vaccines as a global public good. This has yet to be tested. It is also important to consider whether or not such kind of 'altruism' or 'strategic generosity' would be used to deal with future pandemic outbreaks.

China acknowledges the rights of patients to access healthcare as a human right. It also acknowledges that patent rights are very much embedded as rights of holders in the evolution of the modern global political economy. Compared with most developed countries, China is late in coming to terms with both sets of rights. It favours patient rights as development rights (hence, human rights) and increasingly acquires patent rights as it engages with globalisation and competes with other countries over patent filings of industrial inventions and innovation. Within a very short period of time, the country has turned itself from being solely a payer of heavy royalties to also becoming a beneficiary of the patent system. China has begun to pose a significant challenge to prevailing wealthy patent-rights owner-countries like the US and other developed countries in Europe and north-east Asia.

China now needs to strike a delicate balance between the two sets of rights (patient *and* patent), not unlike the dilemma faced by some other countries. The country has shown that it tilts towards favouring patient rights, partly because developing countries, including itself, have suffered so much more historically than developed countries for the lack of patents (and other associated privileges). On the other hand, China has good reasons to champion the cause of making available Covid vaccines as global public goods – a theme we shall return to in our concluding chapter when we discuss the country's newly proposed Global Development Initiative. Before that, let us turn now to examine the rivalries between China and the US in governing global public health – in Chapter 7.

NOTES

1. 'Our world in data: Coronavirus (COVID-19) vaccinations', https://ourworldindata .org/covid-vaccinations#what-share-of-the-population-has-received-at-least-one -dose-of-the-covid-19-vaccine (accessed 27 April 2022).
2. See: https://www.oxfam.org/en/press-releases/covid-19-death-toll-four-times -higher-lower-income-countries-rich-ones (accessed 12 May 2022).
3. See: https://www.hindustantimes.com/cities/pune-news/over-300-covid-variants -may-push-another-wave-of-infection-who-chief-scientist-101666286868303 .html (accessed 22 October 2022).

4.   See: https://www.who.int/about/governance/constitution#:~:text=World%20Health
        %20Assembly%20%C2%BB&text=The%20enjoyment%20of%20the%20highest
        ,belief%2C%20economic%20or%20social%20condition. (accessed 12 May 2022).
5.   See: https:// www .who .int/ news -room/ commentaries/ detail/ health -is -a
        -fundamental-human-right (accessed 12 May 2022).
6.   See: https:// www .mondaq .com/ india/ patent/ 35518/ pharmaceutical -products
        -what -is -not -patentable -under -indian -law #: ~: text = Under %20the %20original
        %20act %20of ,Second %20Amendment)%20Act%20of%202002 (accessed 11
        May 2022).
7.   Rory Horner, 'The world needs pharmaceuticals from China and India to beat
        coronavirus', *The Conversation*, 25 May 2020.
8.   India's many pharma factories and firms 'churn out nearly $50bn-worth of drugs
        a year, accounting for 20 per cent of the world's and 40 per cent of America's
        generics supply by value', *The Economist*, 7 January 2023, p. 54.
9.   *New York Times*, 18 January 2005, quoted in Preet S. Aulakh and Raveendra
        Chittoor, *Coping with global institutional change: a tale of Indian textile and
        pharmaceutical industries* (Cambridge: Cambridge University Press, 2022), p. 1.
10.   Thomas Pogge, 'The Health Impact Fund: how to make new medicines accessi-
        ble to all', in Solomon Benatar and Gillian Brock (eds), *Global health: ethical
        challenges* (Cambridge: Cambridge University Press, 2021), p. 398.
11.   See: https:// www .who .int/ news -room/ commentaries/ detail/ health -is -a
        -fundamental-human-right (accessed 12 May 2022).
12.   Thomas Pogge, 'Just rules for innovative pharmaceuticals', *Philosophies*, 12
        July 2022, p. 14, https://doi.org/10.3390/philosophies7040079.
13.   The idea of patents in this and the following paragraphs is taken from Silvia
        Salazar, 'Intellectual property and the right to health', https:// www .wipo .int/
        edocs/ mdocs/ tk/ en/ wipo_unhchr_ip_pnl_98/ wipo_unhchr_ip_pnl_98_3 .pdf
        (accessed 25 April 2022).
14.   Salazar, 'Intellectual property'.
15.   See: https://www.wto.org/english/tratop_e/trips_e/tripsfacsheet_e.htm (accessed
        26 November 2022).
16.   Kenneth C. Shadlen, Bhaven N. Sampat, and Amy Kapczynski, 'Patents, trade
        and medicines: past, present and future', *Review of International Political
        Economy*, Vol. 27, No. 1 (2020), pp. 75–97.
17.   Salazar, 'Intellectual property'.
18.   TRIPS flexibilities can be seen as 'policy spaces' for countries to mitigate the
        impact of patents, that is, the excessively high price of patented medicines due
        to lack of competition. See https://haiweb.org/wp-content/uploads/2019/06/HAI
        -TRIPS-Brochure.pdf (accessed 26 November 2022).
19.   Medecins sans Frontieres has provided a report discussing these two alternatives;
        see 'Compulsory licenses, the TRIPS waiver and access to Covid-19 medical
        technologies', MSF briefing document, May 2021.
20.   'Parallel import', Wikipedia, https:// en .wikipedia .org/ wiki/ Parallel _import
        (accessed 31 December 2022).
21.   See: https://www.pagewhite.com/news/what-is-a-patent-pool-and-how-does-it
        -operate (accessed 31 December 2022).
22.   This definition is drawn from Olga Gurgula, 'Compulsory licensing vs. the IP
        waiver: what is the best way to end the COVID-19 pandemic?', South Centre,
        Geneva, policy brief, No. 104 (October 2021), p. 2.

23. Cao Zhang et al., 'The legislative approach and system improvement of China's compulsory licensing for drug patents', *Drug Design, Development and Therapy*, Dovepress, No. 15 (2021), p. 3717.

24. Zhang et al., p. 3722.

25. See: https:// www .oxfam .org .nz/ news -media/ pfizer -biontech -and -moderna -making-us1000-profit-every-second/ (accessed 11 May 2022).

26. See: https:// docs .wto .org/ dol2fe/ Pages/ SS/ directdoc .aspx ?filename = q:/ IP/ C/ W669.pdf&Open=True (accessed 12 May 2022).

27. The wide support by developing countries for vaccine equity in the UN context can be seen here: https:// www .un .org/ pga/ 75/ wp -content/ uploads/ sites/ 100/ 2021/03/PGA-letter-The-Political-Declaration-on-Equitable-Global-Access-to -COVID-19-Vaccines.pdf (accessed 23 September 2022).

28. See: https://www.aljazeera.com/opinions/2022/4/8/the-leaked-wto-covid-patent -waiver-text-promises-a-very-bad-deal (accessed 20 April 2023).

29. See: https://www.theguardian.com/world/2021/may/05/us-declares-support-for -patent-waiver-on-covid-19-vaccines (accessed 14 August 2022).

30. Gurgula, 'Compulsory licensing vs. the IP waiver', pp. 5–6.

31. Jane Kelsey, 'Why a leaked WTO "solution" for a COVID patent waiver is unworkable and won't make enough difference for developing countries', *The Conversation*, 21 March 2022.

32. See: https:// www .newsclick .in/ leaked -text -incorporates -stringent -trips -plus -elements-global-calls-rejection-increase (accessed 16 May 2022).

33. See: https://www.riotimesonline .com/ brazil -news/ rio -politics/ brazil -agrees -to -surrender-special-wto-status-for-oecd-entry/ (accessed 14 August 2022).

34. See: https://www.aljazeera.com/opinions/2022/4/8/the-leaked-wto-covid-patent -waiver-text-promises-a-very-bad-deal (accessed 29 August 2023).

35. See: https:// www .reuters .com/ business/ healthcare -pharmaceuticals/ main -negotiators -reach -outcome -covid -vaccine -ip -waiver -wto -2022 -05 -03/ (accessed 13 May 2022).

36. Interestingly, this is the date that China launched its third aircraft carrier.

37. Chinese entities in the process of developing mRNA vaccines include the Academy of Military Sciences, Walvax Biotechnology Co., Ltd., Suzhou Abogen Biosciences Co., Ltd., Shanghai East Hospital, Stemirna Therapeutics Ltd., and Zhuhai Lifanda Biotechnology Co., Ltd. See Huang Zhiming et al, 'Review on drug regulatory science promoting COVID-19 vaccine development in China', *Engineering*, No. 10 (2022), Table 2, p. 130.

38. 'A Chinese mRNA COVID vaccine is approved for the first time – in Indonesia', *Reuters*, 1 October 2022.

39. See: https:// www .reuters .com/ business/ healthcare -pharmaceuticals/ chinas -cansino-confident-its-mrna-covid-vaccine-good-moderna-pfizer-shots-2023-02 -03/ (accessed 26 February 2023).

40. See: https://www.bbc.com/news/world-asia-china-65036474 (accessed 20 April 2023).

41. See: https://www.tandfonline .com/ doi/ full/ 10 .1080/ 21645515 .2022 .2095837 (accessed 14 March 2023).

42. See: https://www.reuters.com/world/china/china-declares-decisive-victory-over -covid-19-2023-02-17/ (accessed 30 April 2023).

43. See: https://edition.cnn.com/2023/04/17/economy/china-gdp-q1-2023-intl-hnk/ index.html (accessed 20 April 2023).

44. China's official forecast was 5 per cent, while the World Bank's was 5.6 per cent and the IMF's 5.2 per cent, as of August 2023.

45. Ou Jiezheng, *Dang zhongyi yushang xiyi [When Chinese medicine meets Western medicine]*, rev edn (Hong Kong: Joint Publishing [H.K.] Co., Ltd., 2023), pp. 278–88. For a report on the contributions of Chinese medicine towards ameliorating Covid, see *Yazhou Zhoukan [Asiaweek]*, Hong Kong, 30 March–5 April 2020, p. 29.

46. I have developed this concept of geo-developmentalism in my previous works. See my trilogy of China's BRI published by Edward Elgar Publishing: *Understanding China's new diplomacy: Silk Roads and bullet trains* (2018); *China's maritime Silk Road: advancing global development?* (2020); and *China's digital Silk Road: setting standards, powering growth* (2022).

47. See: http:// hrlibrary .umn .edu/ research/ ratification -china .html (accessed 15 August 2023).

48. 'Development of China's public health as an essential element of human rights', White Paper, Information Office, State Council, September 2017, Preface.

49. See: https://www.ncbi.nlm.nih.gov/pmc/articles/PMC7989297/ (accessed 5 September 2022).

50. See: https://www .ncbi .nlm .nih .gov/ pmc/ articles/ PMC7989297/ (accessed 5 September 2022).

51. The discussions from Tables 6.1 to 6.3 are largely sourced and updated from my *China's digital Silk Road: setting standards, powering growth* (Cheltenham, UK, and Northampton, MA, USA, 2022), pp. 55–57.

52. 'China's 5G buildout on track after being slowed by Covid-19 outbreak', *South China Morning Post*, Hong Kong, 26 May 2020, p. 16.

53. For a comparative view of the IP filings of some major countries from 1883 to 2019, see *World intellectual property indicators 2020* (Geneva: WIPO, 2020), p. 14.

54. Jiang Renai et al., 'Measuring China's international technology catchup', *Journal of Contemporary China*, Vol. 29, No. 124 (2020), p. 523.

55. 'Why China's intellectual property protection matters to Beijing and Washington', *South China Morning Post*, internet ed., 5 May 2021.

56. 'Why China's intellectual property'.

57. *World intellectual property indicators 2019* (Geneva: World Intellectual Property Organization, 2019), p. 15.

58. *World intellectual property indicators 2019*, p. 18.

59. *World intellectual property indicators 2020*, p. 20.

60. See: https:// www .iam -media .com/ article/ switzerland -once -again -named -the -worlds-most-innovative-country (accessed 2 November 2022).

61. See: https:// wiki .clicklaw .bc .ca/ index .php ?title=Trademarks,_Copyright_and _Other_Intellectual_Property#:~:text=A%20patent%20protects%20new%2C %20useful,services%20from%20those%20of%20others. (accessed 27 February 2023).

62. 'Patent law of China', Wikipedia, https://en.wikipedia.org/wiki/Patent_law_of _China#:~:text=In%20cases%20of%20joint%20patentees,has%20more%20non %2Dpatentable%20matters (accessed 13 May 2022, author updated).

63. See: https:// www .lexology .com/ library/ detail .aspx ?g = eee6d854 -25c6 -4174 -a697-7cbefb692b0a (accessed 14 May 2022).

64. 'China is taking patents seriously: the world should take notice', *The Diplomat*, 12 December 2019.

65. 'TRIPS flexibilities and access to medicines: a European approach', Health Action International, Amsterdam, n.d., p. 6.

66. See: https://papers.ssrn.com/sol3/papers.cfm?abstract_id=4410986 (accessed 30 April 2023).

67. See: https://www.dovepress.com/the-legislative-approach-and-system-improvement -of-chinas-compulsory-l-peer-reviewed-fulltext-article-DDDT#:~:text=However %2C %20the %20overly %20strict %20regulations ,issued %20in %20China %20so %20far (accessed 16 October 2022).

68. See: https://www.loc.gov/item/global-legal-monitor/2012-04-23/china-measures -for-compulsory-licensing-of-pharmaceuticals-updated/ (accessed 16 October 2022).

7.   Sino–US rivalry: the politics of health

China and the US are the world's two largest economies. Together, they make up 42.5 per cent of global GDP in 2021: the US composes 24 per cent at US$23.32 trillion; and China, 18.5 per cent at US$17.73 trillion.[1] Bilateral trade reached US$600 billion in 2022, an increase over the previous year despite various obstacles[2]: Covid-19, the war in Ukraine, and rising inflation, not to mention bilateral rivalries. China has continued to reap huge surpluses vis-à-vis the US, swelling to a new record of US$404 billion in 2022.[3] This surplus has been a major source of contention between the two countries, especially from the US side, a situation that former President Donald Trump had vowed to change, but to little avail despite the imposition of trade sanctions. Sino–American relations have now fallen to new lows seldom seen since the days of the Cultural Revolution in the 1960s. Has the Biden administration made any difference?

This chapter first looks at how the US views China, and then how China views the US. It examines whether or not the two countries can work together in the area of global health – the focus of this book – which inevitably will affect the rest of the world in dealing with infectious diseases, Covid and beyond.

AMERICA EYES CHINA UNDER BIDEN

In a speech delivered at George Washington University on 26 May 2022, US Secretary of State Antony Blinken summed up America's China policy in three words: invest, align, compete.[4] He points out that the US should *invest* more in the R&D of its home industries, technology, and infrastructure (as China has done in recent years); *align* with its allies and partners to maintain global order and to achieve common (read America-led, Western) objectives; and *compete* with China – a challenger, a rival, a threat – in world affairs. Much can be read into this speech, and many of Blinken's core ideas and objectives have yet to be tested in the coming years.

The US National Security Strategy report, published by the White House on 12 October 2022, used such key words as 'build' and 'modernise'[5] to highlight America's policy towards China and to capture the American drive to achieve similar objectives as invest, align, and compete. In the report, President Joe Biden justifies his policy by pointing out that 'China harbors the intention and, increasingly, the capacity to reshape the international order in favor of one that tilts the global playing field to its benefit'.[6] He continues: 'The PRC is the only competitor with both the intent to reshape the international order and, increasingly, the economic, diplomatic, military, and technological power to do it'.[7] The important point here is that China's increasing capability to compete with the US is posing a major challenge for the latter. Biden says that the coming decade will be crucial for US–China relations.

Clearly, invest and align aims to boost America's power and to strengthen its resolve to compete with China in order to win – with winning competitions in world affairs being the ultimate goal. On the whole, Blinken's speech can be seen as balanced (between the hawks and the doves of American foreign policy towards China); it carries aspirations as well as hope for the country. Above all, America wants to be the winner of this global power contest. Like his commander-in-chief, he recognises that China is the 'most serious long-term challenge to the international order'.

The Chinese Foreign Ministry has refuted such logic, pointing out that China is a 'guardian of the international order'.[8] China, being the disgruntled power in this bilateral interaction, has much more to say in response. In fact, it has a long list of complaints against the US (see the next section). The divergent views of the two superpowers beg the question: Who is challenging or protecting what order? Order, by and large, is a value-laden concept. Different countries usually champion different orders to suit their development. All may not be doom and gloom though, as Blinken also observes that the two countries can 'coexist and cooperate' in areas of common interest. He has cited two specific areas, echoing what Biden had said earlier – namely, climate change and global health. In global health, both China and the US, and probably all other countries too, would like to prevent and prepare for the outbreak of future pandemics, to control the spread of viruses, to minimise the economic and social impacts of diseases, and to exchange information about health emergencies as quickly as possible.

On 20 April 2023, US Treasury Secretary Janet Yellen delivered a speech on US–China economic relations at Johns Hopkins University. She outlined three principles that would guide America's approach to China[9]:

> First, we will secure our national security interests and those of our allies and partners, and we will protect human rights . . .
>
> Second, we seek a healthy economic relationship with China: one that fosters growth and innovation in both countries . . .
>
> Third, we seek cooperation on the urgent global challenges of our day. Since last year's meeting between Presidents Biden and Xi, both countries have agreed to enhance communication around the macroeconomy and cooperation on issues like climate and debt distress.

Based on a literal reading of these three principles, there should be no problems between the two largest economies of the world, but Yellen might have a slightly different take on how to manage Sino–US relations compared with her colleagues in the Pentagon and the National Security Council. The critical point of difference is how the US interprets its national security interests and how it perceives the extent of threats it faces. Has China harboured intentions to threaten the national security interests of the US?

CHINA EYES AMERICA UNDER XI

It takes two to tango. What then is China's view on Sino–American relations? At a meeting between Chinese Foreign Minister Wang Yi and his counterpart Antony Blinken on the sidelines of the G20 foreign ministers' meeting held in Bali, Indonesia, in July 2022, China put forward its views. The country emphasised several points which it sees as necessary to overcome the current stalemate in bilateral relations. The media have referred to them as the four lists – or more precisely, three demands and one proposal[10]:

- A list of American wrongdoings that must stop;
- A list of key individual cases that the US must resolve;
- A list of bills in the 117th Congress of high concern to China; and
- A list of eight areas of cooperation, including climate change, public health, and people-to-people exchanges.

Details of these four lists have yet to be made public. A Chinese spokesman, Wang Wenbin, however, said shortly after the Wang–Blinken meeting that the lists 'demonstrate China's serious position that the US must stop exercising containment and suppression, stop interfering in China's internal affairs, and stop undermining China's sovereignty, security, and development interests'.[11] The spokesman expressed that China was willing to cooperate with the US based on 'mutual respect, equality, and mutual benefits'.[12]

Wang Yi and Antony Blinken met again on the sidelines of the UN General Assembly in New York in September 2022. Wang reiterated the basis of cooperation should be 'mutual respect, peaceful coexistence, and win–win'.[13] Commenting on the meeting, *China Daily* stressed that both sides needed healthy competition that would bring out the best of each, not competition that aimed to bring about the demise of the other.[14]

The in-person meeting between Biden and Xi, for the first time in their roles as presidents, at the G20 summit in Bali in 2022 offered some hope. The two leaders appeared relaxed and receptive of each other before the cameras. They agreed on some issues on what some political observers have called the '3R' bottom lines: *re-establish* a baseline of in-person, leader-led communications;

re-start senior-official-level dialogues; and *re-assure* the other side of one's strategic intentions so as to lower the level of mistrust.[15] These three Rs seem very basic. Whether or not they can lead to anything substantial in the future, time will tell.

In the meantime, other events have intervened. For example, the balloon incident in early February 2023 led Secretary of State Blinken to cancel his planned visit to Beijing. Russia's war in Ukraine is likely to continue to sharpen Sino–US differences. On the other hand, China's 12-point peace plan,[16] announced in late February 2023 to settle the Ukraine crisis, may offer some opportunities for global conversations. The meeting of the three leaders of the AUKUS pact in San Diego, California, in March 2023 announcing a US$245 billion deal to sell US and UK nuclear-powered submarines to Australia over the next three decades cited the threat of China.[17] (More on AUKUS later.) The Shangri-La Dialogue held in Singapore in early June 2023 among defence ministers of the Asia-Pacific does not seem to have proffered anything new or substantive to ease tensions. Blinken's visit to Beijing eventually took place in June 2023, after three years of Covid closures on both sides. The visits of Treasury Secretary Yellen and climate envoy John Kerry to China came shortly after in July. This was followed by Commerce Secretary Gina Raimondo in August, whose visit was an effort to try to improve ties. Both sides said the discussions were constructive, but these high-level visits do not seem to have resulted in any major breakthroughs. They have only demonstrated how fragile Sino–US relations can be, revealing the deep mistrust and long-term structural differences between the two countries.

STRUCTURAL CONFLICTS BETWEEN CHINA AND THE US

The recent encounters between the top leaders of the two superpowers reveal only the tips of the problems besetting them. Those problems are deep-rooted. The two countries differ not only in their political and economic systems, but also socially, culturally, and ideologically. Bilateral relations have gone through many ups and downs since American independence in 1776. Their early contacts were less than cordial, especially from China's standpoint. The US came knocking on its door for trade in the 19th century and joined European imperial powers to carve up China into colonial possessions during the late Qing dynasty. The overthrow of Qing and its replacement by the Republic of China in 1911 saw some improvements in bilateral relations. The establishment of the PRC in Beijing in 1949 pushed the government of the Republic of China to the island of Taiwan. Bilateral relations quickly turned sour, heightened by the Korean War of 1950–53. From then on, the containment of Chinese communism and the support of Taiwan worsened relations, just short of going to war. The Mao Zedong years witnessed a period of intense Cold War rivalries between the two until rapprochement came in the early 1970s. Richard Nixon's seven-day visit to China in February 1972 was described by historians as 'the week that changed the world'.[18] The two countries found reasons to work together to counter the Soviet Union in the big power triangle. Deng Xiaoping's reform and opening up of China led to a honeymoon period of bilateral engagement. China began its phenomenal rise in power, first in economics, then in politics and in the military. This changed the balance of power between the two. China's entry into the WTO in 2001 marked a new period of China's rise up to this day.

From 2001 to 2021, the size of China's economy has grown from the sixth largest in the world to the second, and the volume of its trade has risen from the sixth to the largest in the world. It has become the number-one trading partner for more than 140 countries. In 2021 China has established 21 free trade zones around the world, up from zero ten years ago. It has increased its free trade agreements from 10 to 19.[19] China's embrace of globalisation has propelled it to the position of a superpower, especially in economics. In politics, China has been catching up in global influence, especially in the developing world. The only sector where a wide gap still exists is the military: America's high military spending over a long period of time, its numerous military bases and alliances around the world, and its formidable aircraft carrier groups are unparalleled in human history.

The US, however, has started to feel increasingly uncomfortable and worried, as its leadership position in the world is being challenged. The perception of a 'China threat' has become real. Xi Jinping's assertive response, seen by some as aggressive and others as uncompromising, and Joe Biden's continuing to put pressure on China in various ways plummeted bilateral relations to new lows. Biden has maintained the trade war started by Trump in 2018, and, in some cases, has increased the pressure such as banning the sales of advanced semiconductors to China and adopting more protectionist measures at home, cutting an increasing number of political and economic ties with China. Mutual trust is largely absent.

Since the launch of the BRI in 2013, the US has been highly critical of it, casting doubts over its viability, finding faults in various projects, and exaggerating its weak points, and sometimes attacking it in a sloppy way.[20] Li Mingjiang, a seasoned analyst of Chinese foreign policy and Sino–US relations based in Singapore, has pointed out that[21]:

1. The US has taken a leading role in securitising the BRI, promoting a negative narrative about it in the world, and undermining its popularity and impact;

2. The country has attempted to play an oversight role, unceasingly high-lighting the need for higher standards for BRI projects; and
3. It has made strenuous efforts to come up with its own financial schemes and funding arrangements with its allies with a view to compete with the BRI, the most recent example being the Partnership for Global Infrastructure and Investment.

To Li, there is no doubt that the BRI would continue to be a major source of strategic rivalries between the two.

What has China done to defend itself and to protect its interests in the face of American attacks? First, it has taken retaliatory measures in a tit-for-tat way by imposing tariffs and sanctions on US products. Apparently, these Chinese counter measures are in smaller amounts and in limited scope to allow room for negotiation to deescalate tensions. Internally, China has taken measures to adjust its economy. At a national conference in May 2020, Chinese President Xi said that the country needed a development programme that would 'take the domestic market as the mainstay while letting international and external markets boost each other'.[22] This is an indication of China picking a more self-reliant route to protect its economy from the harm done by US decoupling, especially in cutting the supply chain of hi-tech products. In this way, China has launched its 'dual circulation' economic strategy.

IS DUAL CIRCULATION AN EFFECTIVE CHINESE ANSWER?

The word dual in 'dual circulation'[23] refers to a two-track approach to the running of China's economy: a domestic track of economic circulation and an international one. These two tracks reinforce each other. A proper balance between the two would serve to achieve an optimal outcome of interest max-imisation. If one track is obstructed (in this case, it refers to the international circulation), then the other track should receive greater attention and effort for development. The ultimate goal, then, is to achieve a balance and an overall positive economic growth and sustainability.

In reality, multiple tracks exist along which China works or would work with the West in the current global system. China beats its own path of global development based on various bilateral and multilateral arrangements, part-nering in the main with developing countries to forge an alternative system to soften the impact of Western sanctions. China 'walks on two legs' as it were – harking back to the days of the Great Leap Forward in the 1950s when it advanced a balanced development between agriculture and industry – to maintain a balance so as to achieve an optimal outcome, relying on *both* its domestic drive *as well as* working as cordially as possible with the outside world, in the particular the West, although under severe sanctions and isolation as a result of the Korean War.

These days, China has built up greater confidence to compete with the West. It has scored some successes in its development in the global political economy, in the areas of trade, investment, and finance. The West has become increasingly concerned and worried about China's high sustained growth and, on many occasions, has looked for ways to dampen such growth, including sometimes changing the rules of the game or playing double standards such as the use of industrial policies and state subsidies. In facing such a hostile climate, China has revived its traditional way of beating its own path as a way to continue to develop and modernise. This has led to an increasing reliance on self-help, while keeping the dual approach: not to close off completely to the outside world, unlike Mao's complete self-isolation at the height of the Cultural Revolution in the 1960s.

Self-reliance is not an idea Mao originated, although he had pushed such practice to a new level. The idea and its practice can be traced back to China's earlier contacts with the outside world. For example, when Lord George Macartney, representing King George III of Great Britain, came to knock on China's door in 1793 to demand trade, the Qing emperor Qianlong was reported to have said, in part arrogantly and in part ignorantly, in a reply letter to the King: 'Our Celestial Empire possesses all things in prolific abundance and lacks no product within its own borders. There was therefore no need to import the manufactures of outside barbarians in exchange for our own produce'.[24] In China's early modernisation effort during the late Qing dynasty, there was a popular call among intellectuals to take Chinese learning as the essence and use Western learning as a tool (中学为体、西学为用). This is a dual approach combining Chinese characteristics and the best that can be harnessed from the outside, according to China's calculations. China is demographically a huge country and traditionally an agrarian society: farmers tilling their land often have to rely on themselves for survival, as outside help is often not available or is too far away, so a strong sense of self-help and self-reliance has been built into the Chinese psyche over centuries, a process of social learning.

In general, within the West, some countries have adopted different ways to engage with China. The American approach is sometimes at odds with the European approach, based on their different assumptions and assessments of China's challenge on specific issues at specific times. Within Europe itself, countries in the western part of the continent sometimes take an approach different from those in the central and eastern regions. Even within the western part itself, there are subtle differences too: the French approach is quite different from the British one, for example. Further afield, Australia's approach is quite different from that of Japan's or India's for that matter, although they are all in the Quad led by the US. The common feature among them, however, is that they choose to side largely with the Western camp under the strategic, security, and military leadership of the US. India is somewhat unique: sometimes it plays a balancing act between the West and the East, and sometimes it adopts a largely independent, non-aligned path.[25] Indian's variegated responses to Covid-19, China's BRI, and Russia's invasion of Ukraine serve as good examples. (See also India's policy towards the Indo-Pacific Economic Framework below.)

China has a two-pronged approach to healthcare management too, seemingly in line with its 'dual circulation' approach to economic development. On the one hand, it tries to enhance its healthcare services and raise its health standards at home; on the other, it engages actively with other countries in the Western-dominated system, while proactively developing its own way of global ordering, including the building of relevant functional institutions and the promotion of relevant norms and standards relating to global health. (See the sections on telehealth in Chapter 2 and on China's health assistance to Africa in Chapter 5.) In a bigger picture, China's economic statecraft can be viewed as a kind of mercantilism with Chinese characteristics or a kind of modern Sinocentric trade system. When projecting this feature overseas, it has become what David P. Goldman calls 'Sino-forming' the world, especially the Global South.[26] This means that China has been persuading and/or putting pressure on developing countries to comply with its norms and standards. Figure 7.1 shows, in a simplified form, the paths that China takes to reach out to various parts of the world. Although the duality in dual circulation puts emphasis on the balance between the international circulation and the domestic circulation, the international circulation in fact comprises numerous pathways and is more complex than the monolithic nature that the term might have suggested.

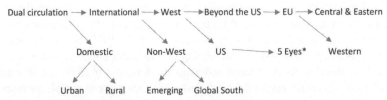

Note: The pathways are non-exclusive and non-linear. They can usefully be visualised as a circular movement in a spiral form. Also, there are interactions and feedbacks among the entities identified in the figure.
*5 Eyes security alliance: AUKUS + Canada and New Zealand.
Source: Author.

Figure 7.1   *Pathways of China's 'dual circulation' statecraft*

'Dual circulation' can be regarded as a newly enhanced version of self-reliance employed by Chinese leaders to adapt to the conditions the country faces and to meet its current development needs. Chairman Mao Zedong emphasised the use of self-reliance in the 1950s and the 1960s to survive on its own resources and capability, due to isolation imposed by big powers – the containment by the US and the West subsequent to the 1950–53 Korean War and then the abandonment by the Soviet Union as a result of an ideological split in the 1960s, leading eventually to a short border skirmish between the two communist powers in 1969. China under Mao had little choice but to rely on its own assets to develop. China's phenomenal economic growth and rapid political rise since the reform and opening up in the 1980s have probably stunned the US and the West. Feeling threatened or unfairly traded or both, President Donald Trump imposed relentless sanctions and boycotts of Chinese goods, reviving in earnest America's strict containment policy of yesteryears. The tightening grip of containment has not been eased under the Biden administration, only to be modified to suit the extant strategic environment and the political climate at home. This has rekindled and renewed China's sense of urgency to return to self-help to deal with the circumstances it faces.

This time around, things are different, as China has become a formidable global power. It is now able to compete more confidently and effectively with the US than before. China's globalising since Deng Xiaoping has served well the country's interests and aspirations. The process of China's increasing interactions with other countries is ongoing with little sign of abating. To China, the outside world is not the global chessboard for big players like the US and the West alone, it is also an arena for the Global South and emerging economies to play a bigger (and fairer) part. As to Sino–US rivalry, China is of the opinion that the world is big enough to accommodate both.[27] There is no good reason for China to withdraw from making connections with the outside world. China can widen its global socialising process, maintaining interactions with the US and the West as much as possible, but also increasing its interactions with the Global South and emerging economies under the BRI and South–South cooperation. In parallel with its increasing international contacts, it also turns inwards to develop its own large and growing domestic market: the internal circulation. This statecraft of dual circulation is much more nuanced, complex, and sophisticated than the policy of self-reliance in the Maoist days.

Domestically, China has realised for several decades since its reform and opening up the importance of balancing developments to narrow the wealth gap between the rich and the poor, between the urban areas and the countryside, and between the east coast and the western part of the country. One of the reasons for initiating the BRI was in fact to help develop the country's underdeveloped west.[28] The HSR, with the extension of its digital healthcare system, would contribute towards helping poorer people in the remote parts of the country to get (better) access to healthcare. These are tools for the central government to achieve the country's goal of common prosperity – a more evenly distributed wealth generated by a more capitalist and innovative sector of the economy. This sector includes the high-tech industry and now the healthcare service. In a curious twist, China uses capitalism as a tool to promote socialism, balancing between the two in its own way under its own conditions.

The ultimate aim of the government seems to be to sustain the country's economic growth and to shield it from the negative impacts of decoupling and other anti-China measures adopted by the US and its allies.[29] Dual circulation is by and large a defensive strategy in response to US pressure. Yet it is a pragmatic way to fend off the tough tariffs and trade sanctions imposed by the outside to stifle the country's growth in general and to cut off its supply chain of critical components like advanced semiconductors to its hi-tech industry in particular. It is a hybrid economic system geared towards striking a balance between external economic exchanges and domestic ones so as to achieve an optimal outcome under trying circumstances. It can be likened to a hybrid car, in which the use of petrol and electricity can either be switched on or off to achieve the best energy efficiency that the car can offer under different driving conditions. It tries to lessen the impact of external political pressure that causes damage to its economy. The goal is to achieve comparative advantage under harsh conditions. Its execution needs to be flexible and fluid. In a way, it can be deployed to work for the benefit of the country rather than leaving the fate of the economy entirely to the whims of the free market, thus challenging the received wisdom that free market is a superior economic model. The free market usually works well for the big, established powers but not so for the weak, the emerging, and the vulnerable. The digital yuan that China is actively developing serves a similar dual purpose: originally designed for internal use, it can be applied externally as a means of international exchange as well. Iran, Russia and Venezuela have increasingly used the yuan to settle the financing of bilateral trade with China instead of the dollar.[30] Saudi Arabia is considering doing something similar. The e-yuan could help to stimulate and sustain China's domestic growth even if its international use is being curtailed.[31]

In the foreseeable future, common prosperity and dual circulation are likely to be the two major features of China's domestic economy, features that carry strong external links. Their practice is highly dependent on the external environment, in particular relations with the US.

IS THE US BENT ON SUPPRESSING CHINA?

Yes, from China's point of view. One of the four Chinese complaints levied at the US centres around the anti-China legislations proposed during the 117th Congress in 2021–22. Known as 'To counter the malign influence and theft perpetuated by the People's Republic of China and the Chinese Communist Party' (or 'Countering Communist China Act', for short), the bill is nearly 300 pages long.[32] It is the most comprehensive and damning bill introduced by the Republican Study Committee in Congress to combat the 'China threat', receiving bipartisan consent.

Among other things, the Act aims to[33]:

- Ban the United Front Work Department of the Chinese Communist Party (CCP) from accessing US financial institutions;
- Prohibit American companies that receive federal subsidies to expand their business in China and affiliate with businesses with ties to the Chinese military;
- Prohibit universities from obtaining grant money from the National Science Foundation to work with entities with ties to the CCP;
- Establish new sanctions on Chinese companies that steal US intellectual property, including prohibiting them from transacting again with a US person;
- Require a determination into whether China's negligence and coverup of the Covid-19 virus would meet the criteria of negligently using a biological weapon; and
- Create a new Select Committee inside Congress to investigate the Covid-19 coverup.

This bill represents by far the most intrusive legislation against China, treating China as the CCP and the CCP as China. It is bound to stir up strong responses and retaliatory actions from the Chinese government, if China's tit-for-tat behaviours in recent times are anything to go by. For the time being at least, the Chinese government would require the US government to take China's concerns seriously before bilateral relations could have a chance to revive. Introduced before the 2022 summer recess of Congress, the bill needs to go through both the House of Representatives and the Senate before being presented to President Biden to sign it into law. It portends to replace previous similar legislation passed that dealt with China in recent years. For example, in early February 2022, the House passed a bill called the 'America Competes Act of 2022' worth US$300 billion to support research on critical technologies, to subsidise the production of computer chips, and to ensure the smooth working of supply chains. The House had to negotiate with the Senate to pin down the bill to be signed into law by the president, which could have taken weeks or months to materialise. The Senate passed its own bill called the 'U.S. Innovation and Competition Act' in mid-2021, worth US$250 billion, to compete with China. America's heavy subsidies to its own industries to boost their competitiveness against China have drawn the ire of European governments for the harmful effects on European companies.

Like many similar bills passed in the US to punish foreign states such as Russia, Iran, North Korea, and many other countries, they are largely unilateral actions. The US, however, also put pressure on allies and close partners to force them to fall into line. Many of these activities rarely go through multilateral processes or international organisations to gain wider international legitimacy. The states at the receiving ends of these actions are the targets of the long (and very strong) arm of US law.

To take a page from these policies, the National People's Congress of China adopted on 28 June 2023 (coming into force on 1 July 2023) the Law on Foreign Relations with the aim to 'safeguard China's sovereignty, national security and development interests (Article 1)'.[34] The law mentions the BRI (Article 26) and the Global Development Initiative, the Global Security Initiative, and the Global Civilisation Initiative (Article 18). Together with the Anti-Foreign Sanctions Law passed in 2021 and the revamped Anti-Espionage Law in effect on 1 July 2023,[35] the new rules form part of Beijing's response to the US-led sanctions that have blacklisted more than 1300 Chinese companies and officials over alleged wrongdoings, including human rights abuses and suspicious ties with Russia.[36] Just as the US has published official reports accusing China of human rights abuses, the Chinese have published their official reports on American human rights abuses, such as US gun laws and police brutality against Black citizens. And just as the US has published its report on China's non-compliance with WTO trade rules, China has responded in kind, publishing its first report in August 2023, titled '2023 Report on WTO Compliance of the United States'.[37] To what extent China's new Law on Foreign Relations can deter the West from taking provocative actions in the future remains to be seen, but enacting such a law has closed a loophole in China's legislation.

While the executive branch of the government (the White House and the State Department, or the President and the Secretary of State) may want to work with China on global public health, the legislative branch, however, wants (to be confirmed when the Countering Communist China Act comes into force) to press on investigating the origins of the Covid-19 virus, apparently based on the premise that it originated in a Wuhan biological lab, an idea that was used by former President Trump to blame China for causing the outbreak and the spread of the virus. He consistently and deliberately called it the Wuhan virus or the China virus instead of Covid-19. So far, as of early 2023, official opinions within the US are divided: while the Department of Energy believes the lab leak hypothesis, opinions in America's intelligence community are not uniform.[38] How to tackle these and other divergent American domestic policy agendas will continue to test the mettle of the Biden administration.

IS THE US 'FORCING' ITS ALLIES TO CONTAIN CHINA?

How successful has the US been in rallying its allies and partners to align with its policy to contain China? To a large extent, it seems that their approach has been working. However, small cracks have started to appear in their solidarity. On alignment, it seems that the US needs to do much more work, mainly as a result of its relative power decline vis-à-vis China and, to some extent, the rest of the world since the end of the Cold War. The pulling out of American troops from the Pacific, the Middle East, and eventually from Afghanistan over recent decades, although sometimes tinkered with readjustments like the return to or 'pivot to Asia' in 2010, are indicative of the slowly declining influence of American imperial power, in the economic and political spheres if not in military power. Allies and partners are perhaps feeling too diplomatically sensitive to express openly their views on this global power shift. America's strongest ally, Britain, has also been on a relative decline, giving way to the rise of the US well before the Second World War.

The sudden and chaotic withdrawal of American (and allied) troops from Afghanistan in August 2021 has left a long shadow over alliance politics. Shortly thereafter, EU Commission President Ursula von der Leyen (former defence minister of Germany) proposed the formation of a common European force that would be less beholden to American unilateral actions.[39] German Chancellor Olaf Scholz's visit to Beijing in early November 2022, shortly after the confirmation of Xi Jinping for a third term as President of China at the 20th CCP Congress, the first leader to do so among the Group of Seven countries, may have signalled Germany's more autonomous action. China observers suggest that Germany (and the EU) is trying to carve out some space for manoeuvre between the two superpowers – China and the US – in the midst of their worsening relations.[40] French President Emmanuel Macron was more vocal. Shortly after his return from a state visit to Beijing in April 2023, he said in an interview with the French media that Europe should be more independent and avoid being dragged into a conflict between the US and China over Taiwan.[41] The European Council on Foreign Relations has recently conducted a survey of Europeans' views on China and the US and their conflict over Taiwan. The poll covers 16 168 respondents from 11 countries.[42] In a report released in June 2023, it shows that Europeans are largely in agreement with President Macron. Seventy-four per cent of those surveyed want Europe to cut its dependence on American security guarantees and invest in its own defence capabilities. Forty-three per cent see China as a 'necessary partner'.[43] America's sometimes unilateral move to 'overstretch'[44] itself and then suddenly withdraw from foreign intervention might have inadvertently unnerved many of its allies and partners. On the other hand, the war in Ukraine has galvanised the West against Russia.

The US forging of an Indo-Pacific region since the 2010s to contain China's increasing influence in the Asian Pacific is being tested from time to time. Most recently, India declined to sign an agreement at the Indo-Pacific Economic Framework meeting held in Los Angeles in September 2022 among 14 countries,[45] saying that the benefits that can be derived from such an involvement were not clear. Apparently, in return for signing an agreement, India would like to gain greater access to the American market which had been ruled out by the US government in the Framework arrangement. (Incidentally, India did not join the Regional Comprehensive Economic Partnership either, a grouping spearheaded by ASEAN countries and China, for fear of losing its domestic market to foreign competitors, among other economic and political considerations.) Vietnam, another participant of the Framework meeting, like India, also expressed the view that the terms of the agreement were not clear.[46] Other participating countries would probably like to see the US take the lead to open up its market (instead of maintaining its protectionist measures taken since the Trump administration, as exemplified by the American withdrawal from the Trans-Pacific Partnership in 2017). This Framework was initiated by President Joe Biden exercising an executive order in May 2022 to form a trade pact with Asian countries focused on four pillars: fair trade; supply chain; clean economy; and infrastructure, taxation and corruption issues.[47] As an executive order, it can be overturned by a new president after the next presidential election in November 2024. To counter the US effort to set up the Framework, China has been arguing for a more inclusive trade arrangement in the region, rather than one that divides nations in the region. In any case, the burgeoning Indo-Pacific arrangement represents another layer in the Liberal International Order underpinned by the comprehensive national strength of the US (see Figure 7.2).

In its effort to contain China, why did the US set up AUKUS when there is already the Quad? What can AUKUS do that the Quad can't? Two points seem to make a distinction between the two. One is that AUKUS brings in the UK to form a tighter English-speaking alliance with the US. (I would call it the 'Eye of Three'.) Another is to bring Australia into the nuclear-capable submarine

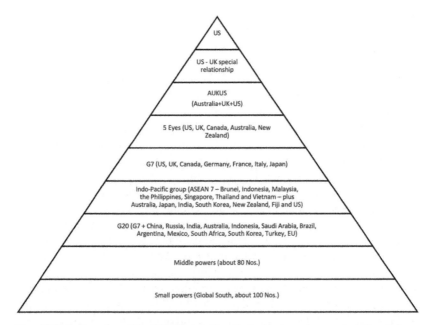

Note: With the formation of the AUKUS pact, New Zealand and, to a lesser extent, Canada have been relegated to play second fiddle to the other three in the 5 Eyes alliance. So have Japan and India in the Quad arrangement in relation to AUKUS. Somewhere at the G7 level, there is a new development of a US–Japan–South Korea alliance.[48]
Source: Slightly modified from Gerald Chan, *China's digital Silk Road: setting standards, powering growth* (Cheltenham, UK, and Northampton, MA, USA: Edward Elgar Publishing, 2022), p. 163.

Figure 7.2   The power structure of the Liberal International Order, 1950–2023

club[49]: the US and the UK announced in 2021 the sale of eight nuclear-powered submarines to Australia while Australia announced the cancellation of its contract to buy a fleet of diesel-powered submarines from France. France was furious: President Emmanuel Macron accused then Australian Prime Minister Scott Morrison of lying and recalled the French ambassador from Canberra. The row was eventually settled by the new Australian Prime Minister Anthony Albanese – an agreement was reached in May 2022 for Australia to pay €555 million (US$585 million) to compensate France, amounting to about 1.5 per cent of the contract price of €35 billion (US$37 billion).[50]

In early March 2023 the three leaders of AUKUS met in San Diego, California, to announce the sales of US and UK nuclear-propelled submarines to Australia at a cost of US$245 billion to be completed by 2055. This will involve the purchase of five US submarines followed by Australia building eight itself with the help of the US and the UK.[51] Although details are still sketchy,[52] the strategic intention seems clear – to combat the 'China threat'. The leaders have planned to rotate American and British nuclear submarines to a naval base in Perth, Western Australia, starting from 2027. An uncertain consequence is the impact on Australia's near neighbour, Indonesia – the most populous Muslim country in the world. In terms of navigation, Australian nuclear submarines would need to go through or near Indonesia's maritime territories in order to move quickly to the South China Sea. The (ill-fated)[53] military exercises held in August 2023 near Darwin, the capital of the Northern Territories of Australia, involving the armed forces of Australia, the US, Indonesia, East Timor, and the Philippines might have in mind the ensuring of a safe and efficient passage of military forces between Australia and the South China Sea. The legal, military, and strategic implications of Australian subs seeking safe passage around Indonesian archipelago waters for military purposes are not entirely clear at this stage.[54] As of March 2023, a senior Indonesian official was quoted as saying that 'the country's sea lanes should not be used by Australian nuclear-propelled submarines because "AUKUS was created for fighting"'.[55]

Apart from the planned naval base in Perth, Australia and the US have beefed up their military alliance by developing a new US airbase in the Northern Territories. The airbase would be able to host six B-52 bombers when completed in late 2026 at a cost of US$100 million.[56] It would be very close to Indonesia and maritime South-East Asia. Geographically, ASEAN countries situate at the heart of the Indo-Pacific region. How would they respond, collectively and individually, to such a new arms race looming in the region?

In February 2023 the US announced that it had reached an agreement with the Philippines to regain its military presence in the country after an absence of 30 years, with expansive access to nine military bases, five currently in use and four new ones.[57] This American military return to the Philippines completes the missing link in the arc of containment of China in the western Pacific Rim stretching from Japan and South Korea in north-east Asia down south to Taiwan and Guam and now to the Philippines and Australia. In May 2023 the US signed a defence agreement with Papua New Guinea to allow American military presence and air and maritime surveillance. This pact helps to tighten further the US encirclement of China.

The small island states in the South Pacific are beginning to express their concerns about the possible nuclearisation of the region, since Australia has decided to acquire nuclear-powered submarines under the AUKUS arrangement. Apparently the AUKUS powers have not consulted the island countries nor the South Pacific Island Forum group as an entity,[58] of which Australia and New Zealand are members. The South Pacific has become a new sphere of competition for influence for the US, Australia, and New Zealand, more collectively than individually, since China's increased presence in the region in recent years.

CAN CHINA AND AMERICA WORK TOGETHER IN GLOBAL HEALTH?

Despite the military tension in the Asia-Pacific, both China and the US have identified healthcare as an area in which they can potentially work together for the benefit of both and others. But how? What can they do?

Some historical context is in order. Bilateral cooperation in healthcare between the two countries started in earnest when they established diplomatic relations in 1979 and when China adopted a reform and opening up policy. Prior to that, some elementary cooperation between academics and medical facilities has taken place since China entered the UN in October 1971 and President Nixon visited China in February 1972, which started a period of Sino–US rapprochement.

In 1978 the US CDC began to explore the possibility of influenza surveillance cooperation with China.[59] A year later the US–China Science and Technology Umbrella Agreement was signed. Exchanges increased in the late 1980s. The first formal agreement was signed in 1989 between the US CDC and the Chinese Institute of Virology. Under the agreement, the US helped the Chinese to set up sentinel surveillance – a network of healthcare providers to collect influenza samples. Once the basic laboratory work was completed in China, all the samples were sent to the US CDC in Atlanta, Georgia, for analysis. Initially the Chinese sent over hundreds of samples a year.

Throughout the 1990s, the US helped China to boost its laboratory capacity and to increase the number of influenza surveillance sites, although the overall scale was still small. In December 2002 the Institute of Virology became part of the newly formed China CDC. In 2008 the China CDC became a WHO Collaborating Center, a status which indicated that China had achieved a certain increased capacity to be able to help other countries to deal with pandemic data sharing, data testing and data analysis. Since then, China's sentinel surveillance (testing people across the community)[60] has grown dramatically, from a handful of sites in the 1980s to 3565 in 2006 and then to 28 685 in 2014.[61] At the same time, the number of laboratories able to run state-of-the-art PCR (polymerase chain reaction) tests (used to detect virus) rose from roughly one in each of China's 31 provinces to almost 400 in the country.[62]

Sino–US relations from the Nixon years in the 1970s to the late Obama years in the 2010s, including the healthcare sector, had largely been amicable. In tackling the bird flu in 1997, SARS in 2002–03, and HIV/AIDS from the 1990s, the working relationships among China, the US, and WHO had been largely cordial. Large-scale disruptions and conflicts had been avoided, despite less than satisfactory results in working together to share information and to trace the origins of disease outbreaks. During the Ebola outbreak in West Africa in 2013–16, both countries sent medical teams to help, answering the WHO's call for international assistance. They even agreed to join efforts to help Africa establish its CDC.[63] (The African CDC HQs are now near completion in Addis Ababa, with sole Chinese funding; see Chapter 5.) Both countries also worked with the African Union to improve healthcare on the continent. The situation started to turn sour in the later years of the Obama administration, and much worse in the Trump years. The outbreak of Covid-19 and the tracing of its origins have become heavily politicised. Working relations during the Trump era had come to a halt, with mutual recriminations – a reflection of the overall frosty bilateral relations.

Much depends on the political will of both sides if meaningful dialogues and cooperation are to resume. There is no lack of good suggestions as to how to make things happen in the healthcare sector. For example, Deborah Seligsohn of Villanova University in Pennsylvania, a specialist in China's healthcare, suggests, among other things, that the US should re-staff its health-related offices in China that had been left vacant, offices such as those of the CDC, the National Institutes of Health, and the FDA.[64] She indicates that both countries have a lot to complement each other in making sure that people around the world are sufficiently vaccinated for Covid-19. Huang Yanzhong and Scott Kennedy, two academics based in the US, have compiled a long list of ways that both countries can work together in the global healthcare field.[65] These range from travel, public health infrastructure, and supply chain resilience to vaccines and therapeutics, biosafety and biosecurity, and countering disinformation. Other observers have also suggested that both countries could work together to help African countries to deal with healthcare issues, like setting up an African Medicines Agency[66] as a specialised agency of the African Union. In general, the US could offer technical support and China could provide health infrastructure and commodities.[67] Why are the two countries not cooperating in combating Covid-19? An analyst in Singapore, Li Xirui, has offered two reasons: one is the ongoing trade and propaganda war between the two countries, which has poisoned bilateral relations; the other is the mismatch in perceptions on how to approach domestic health governance.[68]

The Science and Technology Umbrella Agreement, signed in 1979 when China and the US established diplomatic relations,[69] has served its intended purpose well. Over the past four decades, more than 30 protocols and deals have been signed, and hundreds of joint programmes conducted in many areas, from health and engineering to climate change and environment protection.[70] The Agreement has been renewed about every five years, and the current version is scheduled to expire on 27 August 2023. Nine Republican members of the US House of Representatives, in a letter sent to US Secretary of State

Table 7.1   The divergent global policies of China and the US, 2017–23

	US (under Trump)	China (under Xi)	US (under Biden)
Global approach	De-globalising	Globalising	Re-globalising
Diplomatic practice	Erecting walls, 'burning bridges'	Building roads, bridges, and other connections under the BRI	Build Back Better world; Partnership for Global Infrastructure and Investment
Nature of diplomacy	Protectionist	Opening and inclusive	Still hegemonic?
Global order	Beating retreat	Engaging and reshaping	Reordering
Global power ranking	Falling relatively	Rising relatively	Trying to arrest its fall and suppress China's rise
International relations	Withdrawing	Expanding	Renewing
Political strategy	America First, winner takes all	Geo-economics, win–win	'From relentless war to relentless diplomacy', win–lose
Relations with multilateralism	Denigrating	Embracing, promoting, re-arranging	Returning
Sino–American relations	'Congaging'*; decoupling	More assertive; Tit-for-tat	'Invest, align, compete'; de-risking

Note: * A combination of containing and engaging. Other terms with a similar meaning include limited engaging and conditional engaging.
Source: Slightly modified from Chan, *China's digital Silk Road*, p. 38.

Blinken, said that it should be scrapped because it would enable Beijing to use 'academic researchers, industrial espionage, forced technology transfers, and other tactics to gain an edge in critical technologies, which in turn fuels the People's Liberation Army modernization'.[71] In the absence of any regular and meaningful science and technology exchanges, dialogues, and cooperation between the two governments in recent years, Track II diplomacy has taken over. In the field of healthcare, such a Track II dialogue took place over Zoom in July 2022 between the National Committee on US–China Relations and the National School of Development at Peking University.[72]

Table 7.1 provides a bigger picture of the structural conditions that have helped to shape Sino–US cooperation, including in the field of global health.

China's BRI, of which the HSR is a part, has been referred to in various ways as the country's major, primary, signature, or flagship foreign policy.[73] Without a doubt, it forms the centrepiece of the country's diplomacy. In China's contact with the outside world since the 17th century, it has been largely responding to outside pressures or stimuli – the prying open of China's door by big powers in the West for trade under gunboat diplomacy. This largely one-way flow of influence is now experiencing some sort of reversal:

China is now generating the Grand Stimulus (my terminology) – by promoting the BRI, not by projecting military force or a missionary zeal to help exact unequal trading terms. To refer to China as a new colonialist to developing countries seems an overstretch of historical parallels. To this stimulus, some countries have expressed their welcome and willingness to work with China on various infrastructure projects in order to enhance their national well-being. But there are others who fear China's influence and competitiveness; they have taken steps to contain it or stifle its various initiatives. Then, there are those who choose to sit on the fence, keeping a lookout for good opportunities to make a response. These new stimulus–response interactions have begun to unfold on the world stage.[74] Table 7.2 zooms in on America's responses to this Grand Stimulus. It demonstrates how China's BRI has been exerting a big impact on the behaviour of the US and many other countries.

Is the US playing catch-up in infrastructure building at home and abroad? The US government surely knows that it is falling behind China in advancing development in the Global South. It is, however, still leading in global development overall through various means, bilaterally or multilaterally, as it has done so over a long period of time since the Second World War, but China is starting to narrow the gap between the two in building a new wave of global infrastructure. Facing such a situation, the US chooses a path somewhere between full engagement and full decoupling with respect to China. The swing between these two poles depends on the resultant pull and push of various forces, both domestic and international.

In terms of the BRI, the US is:

- More than ten years behind China in the development of high-speed rail[75];
- About ten years behind in the development of digital currency[76];
- Several years behind in the rolling out of 5G at home[77];
- The International Space Station (launched in 1998) is gradually being phased out in the coming years due to ageing, while the Chinese Tiangong Space Station is just beginning to operate in full force in 2023[78]; and
- China became the top exporter of Covid-19 vaccines in 2021 and is poised to become a global manufacturer of medicines and medical devices (see Chapter 5).

CONCLUSION

In international politics, there is a common saying captured well by Lord Palmerston in his speech before the British House of Commons in 1848: 'We have no eternal allies, and we have no perpetual enemies. Our interests are eternal and perpetual, and those interests it is our duty to follow'.[79]

Table 7.2   China's Grand Stimulus and the US response, 2013–23

	China's Grand Stimulus	US response
Belt and Road Initiative	Trillion-dollar infrastructure projects to connect the world, initiated by Xi Jinping in 2013	Joe Biden proposed a billion-dollar domestic 'Build Back Better' plan in 2021 and launched a G7 US$600 billion 'Partnership for Global Infrastructure and Investment' plan in 2022*
Overland Silk Road	A network of roads, rails, bridges, and power grids across Eurasia and other regions	Yet to start any major projects overseas since withdrawing troops from Iraq in 2007–11 and Afghanistan in 2021
Maritime Silk Road	Consists of three main routes: Traditional route via the Malacca Strait, Indian Ocean and the Red Sea Route to the South Pacific Polar Silk Road	Maintaining military bases and maritime choke points around the world Promoting the Indo-Pacific agenda to contain China Reengaging the South Pacific Initiating its Arctic policy
Digital Silk Road	Digital yuan being rolled out and tested across the country Tiangong Space Station to start full operation in 2023 5G communication widely used across the country	Digital dollar under study, 10 years behind the digitalisation of RMB International Space Station to retire in a few years Rollout of 5G is generally slow and sporadic
Health Silk Road	Vaccine diplomacy: largest Covid-19 vaccine exporter in 2021 Declares Covid-19 vaccines as global public goods Drug production expected to surpass the US in near future	Biden has pledged huge doses of Covid vaccines to poor countries (be)latedly Played a major part in forging the WTO vaccine licensing waiver in 2022 Home to the world's largest pharma companies

Note: * The war in Ukraine would require the US and the West to pour more resources into supporting Kiev. They may therefore find themselves short on reserves to finance major infrastructure projects in developing countries. See 'West follows China's lead with its own "Belt and Roads"', *Asia Times*, https://asiatimes.com/2022/09/west-follows-chinas-lead-with-its-own-belt-and-roads/ (accessed 1 March 2023).
Source: Author.

China and the US have gone through a roller coaster of love–hate relationships from the late Qing dynasty, through the Republic of China, to the
PRC. In the last four decades, China has been rising in global standing and so
posing a challenge, if not a threat, to the US – the current reigning hegemon.
In response, the US has chosen to contain China in order to suppress its rise.
Donald Trump has started the trade war and the propaganda war against China,
and Joe Biden has continued to apply pressure, rallying and reining in allies
and close partners to decouple (later change to de-risk) China in economics
and politics, in trade and supply chains, and in social interactions, citing
national security as the reason. China has responded in kind, but on a smaller
scale, apparently leaving some room for possible de-escalation of conflict.
China has also turned gradually inwards to rely more on itself by adopting
a dual circulation strategy. It has not ceased to promote its flagship diplomacy
– the BRI – only making some adjustments here and there along the way and
initiating new projects such as the Global Development Initiative. To compete
with China and to counter its influence in the developing world, the US and the
other members of G7 have launched the Partnership in Global Infrastructure
and Investment.

How to turn a seemingly destructive competition into a constructive one that
could benefit both as well as other countries? At present, Sino–US relations are
in a quagmire. They seem to be on a long road of rivalry with mutual damage.
Although both countries have indicated that global public health would be an
area in which they could work together,[80] this area, however, has been tied up
with so many zero-sum conflicts. Unless and until cool heads prevail, health
cooperation in America's policy to China would appear to be an afterthought.

NOTES

1. World Bank data, https:// data .worldbank .org/ indicator/ NY .GDP .MKTP .CD
   ?locations=CN (accessed 8 March 2023).
2. 'US and China: whose economy is bigger?', *Business Matters*, BBC World
   Service, 17 January 2023; Statista, https:// www .statista .com/ statistics/
   277679/ total -value -of -us -trade -in -goods -with -china -since -2006/ (accessed
   11 December 2023); also, https://www.bis.doc.gov/index .php/ country -papers/
   2971-2021-statistical-analysis-of-u-s-trade-with-china/file#:~:text=Total%20U
   .S . %20Trade %20in %20Goods , %25 %20(%2445 .0 %20billion) %20increase
   (accessed 17 January 2023).
3. *AP news*, 13 January 2023, https:// apnews .com/ article/ inflation -shanghai
   -business-0c0f7946bc3c08db1df13eb78911f4aa (accessed 14 April 2023).
4. See: https:// edition .cnn .com/ 2022/ 05/ 26/ politics/ blinken -china -speech/ index
   .html (accessed 27 May 2022). The three key words, 'invest, align, compete',
   were reconfirmed by Daniel J. Kritenbrink, US Assistant Secretary of State
   for East Asian and Pacific Affairs, in his keynote speech at the New Zealand
   Institute of International Affairs conference, Auckland, 8 June 2023.

5.   'FACT SHEET: The Biden–Harris Administration's National Security Strategy', The White House, https:// www .whitehouse .gov/ briefing -room/ statements -releases/ 2022/ 10/ 12/ fact -sheet -the -biden -harris -administrations -national -security-strategy/ (accessed 19 October 2022).

6.   'Biden–Harris Administration's National Security Strategy', The White House, https:// www .whitehouse .gov/ wp -content/ uploads/ 2022/ 10/ Biden -Harris -Administrations-National-Security-Strategy-10.2022.pdf (accessed 19 October 2022).

7.   'Biden–Harris Administration's National Security Strategy', p. 23.

8.   See: https://www.cfr.org/timeline/us-china-relations (accessed 6 October 2022).

9.   Full text available in 'Remarks by Secretary of the Treasury Janet L. Yellen on the U.S.–China economic relationship at Johns Hopkins School of Advanced International Studies', US Department of the Treasury, https:// home .treasury .gov/news/press-releases/jy1425 (accessed 22 April 2023).

10. See: https://www.newsweek.com/four-lists-china-wants-us-work-order-improve -ties-1723550 (accessed 30 September 2022).

11. See: https://www.newsweek.com/four-lists-china-wants-us-work-order-improve -ties-1723550 (accessed 30 September 2022).

12. See: https://www.newsweek.com/four-lists-china-wants-us-work-order-improve -ties-1723550 (accessed 30 September 2022).

13. 'Establishing boundaries is essential to ensure healthy, not deadly, competition', *China Daily* editorial, http:// www .chinadaily .com .cn/ a/ 202209/ 25/ WS6330 2e46a310fd2b29e7997c.html (accessed 30 September 2022).

14. 'Establishing boundaries'.

15. 'ICAS TnT dispatch', Institute for China-American Studies, Washington, DC, 2 December 2022.

16. The 12 points can be found at: https:// www .fmprc .gov .cn/ mfa _eng/ zxxx _662805/202302/t20230224_11030713.html (accessed 16 March 2023).

17. 'Australia's nuclear submarine plan to cost up to $245 billion by 2055', *Reuters*, 15 March 2023.

18. See: https://www.wilsoncenter.org/article/the-week-changed-the-world-the-40th -anniversary-president-nixons-china-trip (accessed 16 March 2023).

19. See: https://www.mfa.gov.cn/wjbxw_new/202301/t20230116_11008622.shtml (accessed 20 January 2023).

20. See: https://www .bnnbloomberg .ca/ sloppy -us -talk -on -china -s -threat -worries -some-skeptical-experts-1.1841623 (accessed 27 February 2023).

21. Li Mingjiang, 'The BRI: fuelling strategic rivalry between China and the United States', in Joseph Chinyong Liow, Hong Liu, and Gong Xue (eds), *Research handbook of the Belt and Road Initiative* (Cheltenham, UK, and Northampton, MA, USA: Edward Elgar Publishing, 2021), pp. 416–25.

22. 'Dual circulation', Wikipedia, https:// en .wikipedia .org/ wiki/ Dual_circulation (accessed 26 August 2022).

23. *The Twenty-First Century* bimonthly, published by the Institute of Chinese Studies at the Chinese University of Hong Kong, has published three articles (in Chinese) on 'dual circulation'. See Issue 186, August 2021, pp. 4–45. Also, see Yao Yang, '"Desinification" and China's responses', Issue 180, August 2020, pp. 4–15.

24. See: https:// thechinaproject .com/ 2020/ 09/ 09/ lord -macartney -china -and -the -convenient-lies-of-history/#:~:text=%E2%80%9COur%20Celestial%20Empire

%20possesses %20all ,Lord %20Macartney %20in %20September %201793 (accessed 21 October 2022).

25. Suhasini Haidar, 'Unaligned, non-aligned, or all-aligned? India's foreign policy amidst geopolitical churn', webinar, East–West Center, Honolulu, 7 August 2023.

26. See: https://asiatimes.com/2022/07/sino-forming-of-global-south-passes-point -of-no-return/ (accessed 26 August 2022).

27. Incidentally, US Treasury Secretary Janet Yellen also said, 'We believe the world is big enough for both of our countries to thrive'. She made this remark during her visit to Beijing in July 2023. *South China Morning Post*, Hong Kong, 10 July 2023, p. 1.

28. Gerald Chan, *Understanding China's new diplomacy: Silk Roads and bullet trains* (Cheltenham, UK, and Northampton, MA, USA: Edward Elgar Publishing, 2018), p. 9.

29. The following few paragraphs are sourced from Gerald Chan, *China's digital Silk Road: setting standards, powering growth* (Cheltenham, UK, and Northampton, MA, USA: Edward Elgar Publishing, 2022), Conclusion, with modifications.

30. See: https://www.energyintel.com/00000186-3aad-d94d-a19e-bbedc2700004 (accessed 28 February 2023).

31. Gerald Chan, *China's digital Silk Road: setting standards, powering growth* (Cheltenham, UK, and Northampton, MA, USA: Edward Elgar Publishing, 2022), chapter 5, pp. 66–90.

32. A full text can be viewed at: https://www.congress.gov/bill/117th-congress/ house-bill/4792/text (accessed 5 October 2022).

33. See: https://rsc-banks.house.gov/issue-campaigns/counter-ccp (accessed 5 October 2022).

34. A full text of the law can be found at: http://en.moj.gov.cn/2023-07/11/c _901729.htm#:~:text=Article%204%20The%20People's%20Republic,mutual %20benefit %2C %20and %20peaceful %20coexistence (accessed 16 August 2023).

35. See: https://asia.nikkei.com/Politics/International-relations/US-China-tensions/ U.S.-warns-China-s-new-anti-espionage-law-puts-companies-at-risk (accessed 17 August 2023).

36. 'China unleashes big stick on the legal battlefield', *South China Morning Post*, 10 July 2023, p. A4.

37. '2023 report on U.S. WTO compliance', cgtn.com, https://news.cgtn.com/news/ files/2023-Report-on-U.S.-WTO-Compliance.pdf (accessed 17 August 2023).

38. See: https://www.nytimes.com/2023/02/26/us/politics/china-lab-leak -coronavirus-pandemic.html (accessed 17 March 2023).

39. See: https://www.theguardian.com/world/2021/sep/15/von-der-leyen-eu-state-of -union-speech-political-will-build-own-military (accessed 28 September 2022).

40. 'Silk Road Headlines', *Clingendael*, 11 November 2022.

41. BBC World News, 10 April 2023.

42. See: https://ecfr.eu/publication/keeping-america-close-russia-down-and-china -far-away-how-europeans-navigate-a-competitive-world/ (accessed 13 June 2023).

43. See: https://ecfr.eu/publication/keeping-america-close-russia-down-and-china -far-away-how-europeans-navigate-a-competitive-world/ (accessed 13 June 2023).

44. An idea that Paul Kennedy has popularised to refer to the US involvement in world affairs, in his well-known book, *The rise and fall of the great powers* (New York: Vintage Books, 1989).

45. These 14 countries are the seven ASEAN members – Brunei, Indonesia, Malaysia, the Philippines, Singapore, Thailand, Vietnam – plus Australia, Japan, India, South Korea, New Zealand, Fiji, and the United States.

46. 'Completing the puzzle', *China Report*, July 2022, p. 19.

47. See: https:// www .thenationalnews .com/ business/ economy/ 2022/ 09/ 10/ india -pulls -out -of -us -led -trade -talks -with -asian -nations/ (accessed 26 September 2022).

48. In August 2023 the top leaders of the three countries held a summit at Camp David, just outside Washington, DC. The declared aim was to target military threats from China and North Korea. The Chinese have retorted by saying that this trilateral pact would heighten tensions between rival blocs in Asia.

49. Australia is likely to become the seventh member of this club. See 'Aukus: Australia to pay €555m settlement to French firm', *BBC News*, https://www.bbc .com/news/world-australia-61770012 (accessed 6 November 2022).

50. BBC News, 'Australia is likely'.

51. See: https://www.stuff.co.nz/national/politics/131539796/joe-biden-official-kurt -campbell-says-usnz-agreement-on-cutting-edge-technology-to-come (accessed 19 March 2023).

52. Former Australian prime ministers, Paul Keating and Malcolm Turnbull, have questions about the deal in terms of costs and strategic value. See 'Aukus ruckus leaves NZ sidelined', *Weekend Herald*, Auckland, 18 March 2023, p. A22.

53. The military exercises were called off after an aircraft accident occurred killing three US marines; see: https://www.bloomberg.com/news/articles/2023-08-27/ helicopter -carrying -us -marines -crashes -off -australian -coast -sky #xj4y7vzkg (accessed 30 August 2023).

54. Aristyo Rizka Darmawan, 'Beyond arms race concern: Indonesia and submarine passage in archipelagic waters', S. Rajaratnam School of International Studies, Singapore, IDSS paper, No. 31 (28 March 2023).

55. See: https://www.smh.com.au/ world/ asia/ aukus -created -for -fighting -push -for -indonesia -to -refuse -access -to -subs -20230314 -p5crzz .html (accessed 9 June 2023).

56. 'US B-52 bombers to head to Australia as tensions with China grow', *Radio New Zealand*, 31 October 2022.

57. See: https://theconversation.com/the-us-and-the-philippines-military-agreement -sends-a-warning-to-china-4-key-things-to-know-199159 (accessed 10 February 2023).

58. RTV1, New Zealand, News at Six, 16 April 2023.

59. The narrative of Sino–US cooperation in healthcare in this and the following paragraphs is largely sourced from Deborah Seligsohn, 'The key role of multilateral coordination in the U.S.–China health relationship', in Lucas Myers (ed.), *Essays on China and U.S. policy* (Washington, DC: Wilson Center, 2022), pp. 194–221.

60. According to Wikipedia, sentinel surveillance can be understood as the 'monitoring of rate of occurrence of specific diseases/conditions through a voluntary network of doctors, laboratories and public health departments with a view to assess the stability or change in health levels of a population', https:// en .wikipedia.org/wiki/Sentinel_surveillance (accessed 13 November 2022).

61. Seligsohn, 'The key role', p. 201.

62. Seligsohn, 'The key role', p. 201.
63. See: https:// ustr .gov/ about -us/ policy -offices/ press -office/ fact -sheets/ 2016/ november/us-fact-sheet-27th-us-china-joint (accessed 13 November 2022).
64. Seligsohn, 'The key role', pp. 213–15.
65. Huang Yanzhong and Scott Kennedy, 'Advancing U.S.–China health security cooperation in an era of strategic competition', a report of the Center for Strategic and International Studies Commission on Strengthening America's Health Security, December 2021.
66. A treaty to set up the agency was signed in 2019; see: https://au.int/sites/default/ files/treaties/36892-treaty-0069_-_ama_treaty_e.pdf (accessed 4 January 2023).
67. See: https:// thehill .com/ opinion/ international/ 3609794 -can -the -us -and -china -cooperate-on-african-health-priorities/ (accessed 4 January 2023).
68. 'Why China and the United States aren't cooperating on COVID-19', *East Asia Forum*, https:// www .eastasiaforum .org/ 2021/ 07/ 24/ why -china -and -the -united -states -arent -cooperating -on -covid -19/ #more -371485 (accessed 10 February 2023).
69. 'Future of 44-year-old science agreement caught in middle of U.S.–China tensions', *Axios*, https://www.axios.com/2023/08/05/china-us-tensions-science -technology-agreement-renewal (accessed 17 August 2023).
70. 'Sino–US science deal renewal a stabilizing move', *China Daily*, Hong Kong ed., 30 June 2023, p. 9.
71. 'Sino–US science deal', p. 9.
72. See: https:// en .nsd .pku .edu .cn/ news/ 524862 .htm; https:// www .ncuscr .org/ program/us-china-track-ii-dialogue-healthcare/ (accessed 17 August 2023).
73. This paragraph is a slightly modified version taken from Chan, *China's digital Silk Road*, p. 2.
74. The 'old' stimulus–response relationship has been used as a general framework by John Fairbank of Harvard University to frame China's response to outside stimulus in its interactions with the world.
75. Chan, *Understanding China's new diplomacy: Silk Roads and bullet trains.*
76. Chan, *China's digital Silk Road*, chapter 5.
77. Chan, *China's digital Silk Road*, chapter 5.
78. Chan, *China's digital Silk Road*, chapter 7.
79. See: https:// www .oxfordreference .com/ display/ 10 .1093/ acref/ 9780191826719.001.0001/q-oro-ed4-00008130;jsessionid=AEC36F0D61B5 50A8B6C47E666C28393C (accessed 31 March 2023).
80. Apart from health, climate change is another area of potential cooperation, at least in aiding island countries in the South Pacific from being submerged under rising sea levels.

8. Conclusion

A century ago, George Bernard Shaw, the Irish playwright and Nobel laureate, said that 'the greatest of evils and the worst of crimes is poverty'.[1] To some, 'poverty is a death sentence'.[2] It goes hand in hand with inequality. History has given us ample evidence. More recently, the unequal access to Covid vaccines has resulted in vastly disproportionate suffering by people in the Global South (Chapters 5 and 6). What has the WHO done to tackle the issue of Covid (in) equity? This is the first question that we ask here. Second, what has China done to contribute to global development in general and to the elimination of global poverty in particular? Finally, apart from empirical studies, we bring together the findings in this book by reviewing our theoretical framework – geo-developmentalism – to assess its validity in explaining the workings of the HSR. This assessment can help to reveal some future directions for research in potential change and innovation of global development.

THE WHO AND COVID (IN)EQUITY

On the second anniversary of the WHO's declaration of Covid-19 as a pandemic, 11 March 2023, some 130 leading politicians, activists, and academics signed an open letter to call on state leaders, especially those in the West, to address the issue of unequal access to Covid medicines and to find better ways to deal with future pandemics.[3] At least 7 million people had died as a result of the disease then.[4] In reporting the release of the letter, *Financial Times* of London indicated that 1.3 million fewer people would have died in 2021 had vaccines been distributed more equitably, or one preventable death in every 24 seconds.[5] Ban Ki-moon, the former UN Secretary–General and one of the letter signatories lamented that this 'great tragedy' was due to 'the failure of multilateralism' (or more precisely the failure of cooperation among states in a multilateral setting). The signatories of the letter blamed 'self-defeating nationalism' and pharmaceutical monopolies, apart from inequality, as the sources of this calamity.[6] They argued that Covid vaccines should be regarded as people's vaccines – in other words, a global common good. They called on world leaders to not repeat the same mistakes again in confronting future pandemics.

The WHO is now actively working on a Pandemic Prevention, Preparedness, and Response Accord (or Pandemic Accord for short).[7] The process started in

December 2021. At a special session, the World Health Assembly established an intergovernmental negotiating body to draft and negotiate a convention, agreement, or other international instrument under the Constitution of the WHO to strengthen pandemic prevention, preparedness, and response. In December 2022 a Zero Draft was made, one that is designed for reflection by member states before proceeding to the next stage for discussion and negotiation.

One major proposal in the Zero Draft is that 20 per cent of pandemic-related products such as vaccines, diagnostics, personal protective equipment, and therapeutics should be allocated to the WHO, which would then ensure their equitable distribution. Half of such allocation to the world body (10 per cent of total global production) should be donated, while the other half should be bought at an 'accessible' price.[8] The draft advises poor countries to use flexibilities and the IP waiver as much as possible and suggests that rich countries relax their hold on IPs. The draft is scheduled to go through the intergovernmental negotiating body for discussions and negotiations in 2023. A full draft is scheduled to be tabled in June 2023,[9] and a final draft will be presented to the 2024 World Health Assembly for consideration.[10] The legislative process is likely to go through a tough time, as the US has expressed concerns about possible infringement on its sovereignty. The EU and countries like the UK, Germany, and Switzerland are very jealously guarding their interests in patents and IP. Big pharmaceutical companies in the West have a record of fiercely defending their rights.

Covid-19 has exposed and exacerbated health inequity in the world. According to the IMF, Covid-19 has caused millions of deaths (the official record is 7 million as of early 2023, but unofficial figures are much higher), pushed more than 120 million to extreme poverty, and led to a global recession. It has widened the wealth gap within nations, but even more so between nations. Writing in March 2022 in *Scientific American*, Joseph E. Stiglitz, an economics professor and Nobel laureate, said that 'Global billionaire wealth grew by US$4.4 trillion between 2020 and 2021 [during Covid], and at the same time more than 100 million people fell below the poverty line'.[11]

In September 2022 the UNDP published its Human Development Report, which gives a bleak picture of the current situation of the world: in 2020 and 2021 the world's development slid backwards for the first time since the publication of the report in 1990. The life expectancy of people in 90 per cent of the countries surveyed has gone backwards; so have education levels and the standard of living of the general public. These developmental challenges have been made more acute by climate change and the war in Ukraine, apart from Covid-19. The UNDP suggests three ways to tackle these problems. They are, in short: investment, insurance, and innovation – investment to provide public goods, to prepare for pandemic outbreaks, and to tackle climate change; insurance to cover social protection and to facilitate access to basic human needs; and innovation to span technology, economics, and culture.[12]

The West has experienced centuries of modern development since 1500. In comparison, non-Western countries have undergone only decades of modernisation since 1900; they therefore have to work hard to catch up. They have to push forward their development in a compressed way. Scholars like Chang Kyung-Sup of Seoul National University and D. Hugh Whittaker of Oxford University have used such terms as 'compressed modernity'[13] and 'compressed development',[14] respectively, to describe and explain the rapid development of emerging economies in East Asia, including Japan, South Korea, Taiwan, and China. These countries use state developmentalism as a way to fast-track development, narrowing their wealth gaps with Western countries. China, according to Whittaker, proves to be somewhat unique because of the large scale and fast speed of its development. To him, though, most countries have, in one way or another and at one time or another, gone through some form of compressed development.

The idea of compression can be measured against time and space. Countries undergoing compressed development or compressed modernity face many challenges during the transition, ranging from political, strategic, and economic to institutional, social, and ideological. Very often, they have to make appropriate adjustments to balance tradition and modernity, sometimes through peaceful change, sometimes through violence and revolutions, and sometimes through the use of hybrid measures that lie somewhere between the two.

Having lifted millions of people out of poverty, China has become a model of success for many developing countries to copy. They are drawn to China by joining the BRI – a trillion-dollar development programme that makes connections with countries around the world through the building of infrastructure with the aim of stimulating economic growth based on mutual benefits.

In sum, to tackle global inequality, several measures are needed. These include, among others, development aid, infrastructure building, the provision of public goods, and a fair (re)distribution of wealth. Political will and global effort through multilateral cooperation like the UN system are called for. What has China done to help in this respect?

CHINA ROLLING OUT AMBITIOUS PLANS

The HSR, an extension of China's health diplomacy and a major component of the BRI, has been put through its paces to address the issue of inequality. In January 2023 Deputy Foreign Minister Xie Feng gave a speech on 'China and the World' in a forum held at Renmin University in Beijing. He called on other countries to work with China to develop five areas of common interest[15]:

1. Common development;
2. Common security;
3. Common opening;
4. Common values; and
5. Common responsibilities.

His proposal echoes what top Chinese leaders have been calling for in recent years to address global problems of development, security, and civilisational understanding. Eight years after the launch of the BRI, China has rolled out further initiatives, first the GDI. In a video address to the UN General Assembly in September 2021, President Xi Jinping announced the launch of this initiative. He said it was high time to steer global development to scale new heights that are balanced, coordinated, and inclusive, especially when countries around the world are facing great shocks caused by Covid-19. He stressed the importance of green, innovative, and sustainable development, in line with the aspirations of the UN 2030 Agenda for Sustainable Development and also in response to Western criticisms of China's low-quality construction projects. Xi suggested that the new priorities should include poverty alleviation, food security, Covid-19 response and vaccines, development financing, climate change, industrialisation, the digital economy, and connectivity.[16]

This new initiative has received positive responses from the UN and many developing countries. In January 2022 China's Permanent Mission to the UN launched a drive to form the Group of Friends of the GDI to strengthen policy dialogue, share best practices, and promote project cooperation. The launch event attracted 24 leaders of UN agencies and representatives from over 100 countries.[17] As of mid-2023, close to 70 countries have joined the Group of Friends.[18]

The GDI has been well received by developing countries, including a large number of those in South-East Asia. The reasons why the initiative has been so well received say something about the dire need for infrastructure construction in the countries involved. Hoang Thi Ha, a researcher at the Yusof Ishak Institute in Singapore, has offered some explanations.[19] First, there is a commonly felt need for development. Countries in South-East Asia are now experiencing a development deficiency. To them, the 'right to development' is paramount. This urgent need for substantive infrastructure development has been pointed out by many international financial institutions, including the Asian Development Bank and the World Bank.[20] Second, South-East Asian countries are comfortable with a state-centric approach to development, echoing the state developmental approach to growth adopted by Japan, South

Korea, Taiwan, and China. Third, they share a common worry that the war in Ukraine has diverted significant resources from the West, leaving a diminishing amount for helping the global poor. Many countries in South-East Asia are more concerned with bread-and-butter issues than with matters of high politics, at least for the time being.

Like many bold Chinese initiatives when first announced, the GDI is broad in scope and general in its terms of reference. It contains plenty of broad aspirations, principles, and suggestions. Details are few and far between. According to Chinese initiators, like-minded stakeholders have to work out in finer details what exactly they want and how they would like to move forward together, in big or small groups, to achieve their common goals when the time is right. There are lots of possibilities and flexibilities at this initial stage.

Covid-19 has certainly set back many of the meagre economic achievements made by the world's poor countries prior to the outbreak of the pandemic. The goals set by the UN Agenda for 2030 Sustainable Development are now understood to be hard to achieve, so China's GDI comes in good time to help reboot global development and rebuild momentum to achieve the UN SDGs or at least to narrow as much as possible the gap between targets and actual achievements made so far. A midterm review of the SDGs took place in September 2023. The Secretary-General of the UN, António Guterres, encouraged member states to take united, accelerated action to achieve the SDGs.[21] Apart from China's programmes and efforts, those made by the West and the Global South could be used to make assessments of progress made so far and to chart the way forward for the world's development as a whole.

While the BRI has focused initially on huge infrastructure projects, funded mostly by China's policy banks and built by its state-owned construction companies, with input from host countries where contracted, many of these projects are mounted based on China's bilateral agreements with the host countries. Although the parameters of the GDI are still vague, it seems to have focused more on multilateral cooperation and on 'small and smart' or 'small but beautiful' projects in alignment with the UN SDGs. China intends to act as a coordinator (through the China International Development Cooperation Agency, which was founded in 2018 and falls directly under the control of the State Council) rather than as proprietor of these projects. In a way, the GDI can be seen as a new extension of the BRI rather than its partial replacement. Like the BRI, the GDI is not entirely an aid programme, although some aid elements are likely to be involved. Both can be seen as government initiatives based on corporate involvement and management. The major differences are in the scale and scope of projects, the risks involved, the viability of these projects, and the number of stakeholders.

According to a report by Fudan University's Green Finance and Development Centre, China's Belt and Road Projects rebounded in the first half of 2023. The initiative appears to have regained momentum after the Covid-19 pandemic had slowed its activities for three years. A total of 103 deals worth US$43.3 billion were signed in the first six months of 2023 compared with US$35 billion in the same period the year before. The average value of the deals dropped from US$617 million in 2022 to US$392 million in 2023.[22]

The GDI has been followed shortly by two other initiatives: one focusing on security and the other on cultural exchange; they are, respectively, called the Global Security Initiative (GSI) and the Global Civilisation Initiative (GCI). These three initiatives form a kind of tripartite structure of China's global aspirations and its worldview. Together, they represent a more comprehensive vision and agenda than individually (Figure 8.1 and Table 8.1).

Table 8.1   *Comparing China's three global initiatives: GDI, GSI, GCI (August 2023)*

	Global Development Initiative (GDI)	Global Security Initiative (GSI)	Global Civilisation Initiative (GCI)
When initiated	September 2021	April 2022	March 2023
Where announced	UN General Assembly (online)	Bo'ao Forum for Asia	Dialogue of World Political Parties (online)
Aim/Goal	To reduce poverty through growth and development	To eliminate root causes of international conflicts; improve global security governance[a]	To eschew civilisation clash; respect diversity; promote common values; 'Asian values' back?[b]
Mechanism	Group of Friends of GDI (70 countries)	SCO; CICA; various regional forums in Asia, Africa, and Latin America	UNESCO
China's coordinating agency	China International Development Cooperation Agency	Ministry of Foreign Affairs	Chinese Communist Party
Funding	$4 bn Global Development and South–South Cooperation Fund	Data unavailable	Data unavailable
No. of interested parties[c]	100 countries and organisations	80 countries and organisations	Online dialogue brought together 500 leaders from 150 countries

	Global Development Initiative (GDI)	Global Security Initiative (GSI)	Global Civilisation Initiative (GCI)
Nature	Multilateral; linked to UN SDGs 2030; small and quality projects	Multilateral among developing countries	Multilateral among the non-West and the rest
No. of projects	Initial list of 50[d]	Iran/Saudi Arabia rapprochement cited as an example	Numerous soft power projects

Notes: SCO: Shanghai Cooperation Organisation.

CICA: Conference on Interaction and Confidence-Building Measures in Asia.

[a] See: 'China's role in the Middle East – Jin Liangxiang', *CHINA US Focus* (accessed 23 June 2023); http://gd.china-embassy.gov.cn/eng/zxhd_1/202305/t20230505_11071292.htm (accessed 30 August 2023).

[b] See: https://fulcrum.sg/the-global-civilisation-initiative-are-asian-values-back-with-a-chinese -vengeance/ (accessed 4 May 2023).

[c] In comparison, 150 countries and 32 international organisations had signed more than 200 cooperation documents to work together under the BRI at the end of 2022. The relationship between the BRI and the three global initiatives here can be seen as compatible, complementary, and mutually reinforcing.

[d] A full list can be found at: 中华人民共和国中华人民共和国中, https://www.fmprc.gov.cn/ mfa_eng/wjb_663304/wjbz_663308/activities_663312/202209/P020220921624707087888.pdf (accessed 17 April 2023).

Sources: Various online sources.[23]

This Chinese tripartite approach to global development is different from Western priorities, but it seems to strike a chord with many countries in the Global South. The three major components take economic growth as the keystone to promote modernisation, to enhance mutual understanding across cultures and traditions, and to achieve security based on common, comprehensive, and shared values. The Western worldview, especially that of the US, pays relatively little attention to developmental growth and civilisational understanding, for some understandable reasons, perhaps: the US is already *the* superpower that has been building up its might over a century to now be in a position to exercise and maintain global order and dominance. Its view of security is very much based on a sharp but narrow absolutist view – America First – and on a system of hegemonic, hierarchical structuring and ordering backed by an overwhelming military force. To sustain its current position and to counter China's rise in influence, it has taken an 'integrative deterrence' approach,[24] a deterrence that is increasingly comprehensive and gripping.

In proposing the GDI, China has shown the softer side of its infrastructure approach. This softer side embraces image building, the exercising of soft power, and the displaying of global responsibility. At this early stage, much discussion on the GDI is still focused on policies and ideas. Tying up the goals of its initiatives with that of the UN SDGs has shown China's preference for multilateralism, especially through the UN, and a desire to win over the

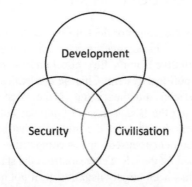

Figure 8.1   *Visualising China's three global initiatives: development, security, civilisation*

support of others, mostly low-income countries, so as to work together in a large-majority group of like-minded countries for common development and mutual benefit.

In sum, China now pursues a global policy that is development-led, buttressed by a shared understanding of national security among countries in the Global South. This is a major contrast to the policy of the US, its main strategic rival in global affairs. The US has nurtured a military-industrial complex over many decades, a system built upon the hegemonic control of the global order and the maintenance of American primacy.[25] It hangs on to a unipolar world in which it is the superpower writ large, against the backdrop of a changing world that is increasingly multipolar in nature, with the rise of China and other emerging economies.[26] This is in essence the crux of the superpower rivalry between China (on relative rise) and the US (in relative decline). China's worldview has offered an alternative global order, one that is based on an old and established system but updated to reflect increasingly China's evolving preferences and values. In this evolving global system, many countries are being forced, willy-nilly, to choose sides. However, some countries are able to make good use of this hard choice to play a smart game of balance of power to optimise their own national interests. Recent examples include Saudi Arabia and the United Arab Emirates.[27] Both oil-rich countries see opportunity where others see risk amid an era of shifting global dynamics. Both want to befriend the two superpowers.

RETHINKING GEO-DEVELOPMENTALISM

Theorising the BRI is not easy, nor does it seem appealing. It is not appealing because, evidently, the Chinese government is much more concerned with the playing out of the initiative than the theoretical understanding of it. Labouring under the country's political system, Chinese academics have relatively little room for free expression and theorising, in the Western understanding of those terms. Theorising the BRI is not very popular outside of China either, due largely to the negative view of the initiative that has been generated in a geopolitical environment focused on the competition and rivalry between China and the West led by the US. Ten years from the start of the BRI in 2013, the US government has been largely negative of, if not hostile to, the Chinese initiative.

Theorising BRI is difficult as the initiative is still relatively new and ongoing. The initiative is so big, involving so many different issues at so many governing levels in so many countries and regions of the world. Different observers and analysts naturally hold different views of this behemoth programme. Under such circumstances, the effort to theorise can be likened to the blind men touching different parts of the elephant, as depicted in the Indian fable, and so coming away with different understandings of what an elephant looks like.

The fact that it is difficult and unpopular to theorise has not prevented scholars from attempting to do so, although efforts have been few and far between. Some use a geopolitical approach, others use a mercantilist approach, while still others use political economy, globalisation, state capitalism, and myriad other theories and sub-theories. I have tried to use an idea I call geo-developmentalism to capture the essence of the BRI. The idea has evolved into a concept and a framework for analysis. I sometimes use the word theory to describe this idea, but I shy away from referring to it as a theory in a very strict sense of the word in social sciences, with great ability to explain causal relationships and to help predict future developments.

Geo-developmentalism is an idea that I find interesting and useful, as it captures well the element of the geographic spread of China's state developmental approach to the global political economy. It came to light when I was intrigued by the One Belt, One Road initiative that China proposed in 2013. I endeavoured to define the idea with some conceptual trappings in my first book on China's BRI, published in 2018. For the sake of repetition, I have defined geo-developmentalism as: 'China-initiated developmental trajectory of infrastructure building aimed at promoting mutual economic growth by increasing connections across the globe'.[28]

I have identified ten features that characterise the BRI, including constructing infrastructure, the balance between geopolitics and geo-economics, and a win–win outcome for China and partner countries in joint infrastructure building. I have since maintained the integrity of the definition and, since 2018, tried to elaborate in greater detail some of the features of geo-developmentalism. I have also extended the idea to reach out to new developments in International Political Economy (IPE) to propose the emergence of neo-globalisation and neo-transnationalism, especially in view of China's contributions to the theory and practice of IPE and global development.

Is the idea of geo-developmentalism unique to China? Over recent years, the BRI has attracted a lot of attention, and many countries have started their own infrastructure development, partly out of their own needs and partly in competition with China. Different countries have adopted different names to label their own infrastructure programmes.

I have highlighted geo-developmentalism as China-led. To me it still holds true, but this Chinese initiative has attracted strong and capable competitors like the United States to put forward possibly better alternatives such as the Build Back Better plan and the Partnership for Global Infrastructure and Investment. The EU too has proposed its Global Gateway. This development only shows the growing currency of geo-developmentalism in the world and its increasing policy impact. China still leads in global infrastructure building, but there is more than enough room for others to play, either working with China or independently. Thus global infrastructure development, initially started by China on a vast scale, has moved to engulf the policy space and practice of many other countries, friends and foes alike, and others in between. Global infrastructure development has become a new global norm. The idea of geo-developmentalism, which embraces infrastructure development at its core, acknowledges China's contributions to global development and international relations. Other countries have accepted or rejected it based on their different calculations of national interest.

The interesting and challenging aspect of trying to theorise the BRI is that it is not something static. Rather, it is something moving, and moving rapidly, despite the disruption caused by Covid-19 and other events. Also, it evolves. Theorising BRI therefore requires revisions and updates from time to time, using new evidence to continuously test the extant theoretical framing of it. The evidence may support and confirm the existing body of knowledge. Some might refute it or parts of it. A case in point is the new initiatives that China has started, like the GDI, GSI, and GCI. These three new initiatives have the potential to boost the development of the BRI, including the HSR. Depending on the development of these three initiatives in the future, they tend to support and enhance rather than to replace existing projects under the BRI. In terms of better theorising, it is likely that the BRI and the other initiatives will morph into a complex programme of greater scope and increasing legitimacy, becoming acceptable to more countries, especially those in the Global South if not in the Global North. China may then play a greater role in global leadership, helping to define a new world order in its favour.

In the meantime, a major feature of the BRI related to China's balancing between geo-economics and geopolitics is shifting. The country started with putting greater emphasis on geo-economics, focusing on trade, investment, and finance when building infrastructure at home and abroad. But gradually it has shifted to pay greater attention to geopolitics, partly because of the fragile political situation of many host countries and partly because of the political pressure exerted by the US and some Western countries on China, sanctioning trade and decoupling supply chains. This shift on China's part is currently in progress, and its magnitude depends on the extent of external pressure and the specific circumstances involved.

Although China's global development efforts have received negative feedback from many quarters in the West, they have received encouraging support from some major international organisations. A recent example in relation to the HSR is President Xi Jinping's declaration of Covid vaccines as global public goods in May 2020. In a speech made in Paris in November 2020, the Director-General of the WHO, Tedros Adhanom Ghebreyesus, endorsed the idea of treating Covid vaccines, diagnostics, and therapeutics as global public goods.[29] IMF Managing Director Kristalina Georgieva also said in January 2022 that 'it is increasingly clear that a robust and reliable vaccine capacity in Africa is a global public good that deserves global support'.[30] In a way, China's linking of its developmental goals with those of the UN SDGs is a move that has received a positive reception from many developing countries.

CONCLUSION

Developing countries in the Global South are eager to receive global public goods, whether they are coming from neoliberal states that have provided the political economic architecture for global development since the end of the Second World War, or more recently from emerging economies including China. China's three initiatives – GDI, GSI, and GCI – have great potential to help developing countries based on shared responsibility, working together to achieve some common goals in an incremental manner, and legitimisation by the UN's involvement.

Will this new development lead to some structural changes to the existing world order? The answer is yes. Although the Western-dominated liberal international order is still very much in place, a complementary yet alternative China-led order is emerging. There are also other smaller, regional orders in the making. The world seems to be evolving into a multiplex structure, as has been envisioned by some scholars, including one of its advocates, Amitav Acharya.[31] In this multiplex world, China has been changing itself to change the world, connecting itself to connect the world, digitising itself to digitise the world, and developing itself to develop the world.

NOTES

1. See: https://www.azquotes.com/quote/557025 (accessed 20 March 2023).
2. See: https://www.cbsnews.com/news/why-is-bernie-sanders-suddenly-talking-about-poverty/ (accessed 12 May 2023); 'Capital in the twenty-first century', 2019, https://www.nzfilm.co.nz/films/capital-twenty-first-century (accessed 30 August 2023).
3. The full letter is here: 'PVA letter calling for a people's vaccine against COVID-19', https://peoplesvaccine.org/wp-content/uploads/2022/03/Vaccine-Open-Letter-March-2022.pdf (accessed 20 March 2023).
4. Johns Hopkins University data, https://coronavirus.jhu.edu/map.html (accessed 20 March 2023).
5. See: https://www.ft.com/content/fcddc944-5112-4e32-be22-6ead2bc06cc7 (accessed 12 March 2023).
6. 'Call for vaccine equity so COVID "mistakes" are not repeated', 11 March 2023, https://www.dw.com/en/call-for-vaccine-equity-so-covid-mistakes-are-not-repeated/a-64953592 (accessed 20 March 2023).
7. See: https://www.who.int/news-room/questions-and-answers/item/pandemic-prevention--preparedness-and-response-accord (accessed 20 March 2023).
8. See: https://healthpolicy-watch.news/pandemic-treaty-zero-draft-proposes-who-gets-20-of-products/ (accessed 20 March 2023).
9. See: https://apps.who.int/gb/inb/pdf_files/inb4/A_INB4_4-en.pdf (accessed 21 March 2023).
10. See: https://healthpolicy-watch.news/pandemic-treaty-zero-draft-proposes-who-gets-20-of-products/ (accessed 20 March 2023).
11. See: https://www.scientificamerican.com/article/covid-has-made-global-inequality-much-worse/ (accessed 21 April 2023).
12. *Human development report 2021/2022* (New York: UNDP, 2022), pp. 5, 18.
13. Chang Kyung-Sup, *The logics of compressed modernity* (Cambridge: Polity, 2022).
14. D. Hugh Whittaker et al., *Compressed development: time and timing in economic and social development* (Oxford: Oxford University Press, 2020).
15. See: http://rdcy.ruc.edu.cn/zw/qsyj/2023hgxslt/ztlbhglt/ec4cf004cb9445179e4f1429c50a6eb6.htm (accessed 20 January 2023).
16. 'Xi proposes Global Development Initiative', *Global Times*, 22 September 2021, https://www.globaltimes.cn/page/202109/1234780.shtml (accessed 12 December 2023).
17. 'Group of friends of Global Development Initiative launched', *Xinhua*, 21 January 2022, https://english.news.cn/20220121/81050f6ae91e49bc8e0b019f4eabb1d0/c.html (accessed 12 December 2023).
18. See: https://global.chinadaily.com.cn/a/202306/20/WS6490d47ba310bf8a75d6abdf.html (accessed 18 August 2023).

19. 'Microsoft Word – ISEAS_Perspective_2023_9', https://www.iseas.edu.sg/wp -content/uploads/2023/01/ISEAS_Perspective_2023_9.pdf (accessed 23 March 2023).

20. Gerald Chan, *Understanding China's new diplomacy: Silk Roads and bullet trains* (Cheltenham, UK, and Northampton, MA, USA: Edward Elgar Publishing, 2018), p. 14.

21. See: https:// www .un .org/ en/ conferences/ SDGSummit2023 (accessed 11 December 2023).

22. 'China's Belt and Road Initiative regains momentum as focus shifts to smaller "high-quality" projects', *South China Morning Post*, https:// www .scmp .com/ news/ china/ diplomacy/ article/ 3230094/ chinas -belt -and -road -initiative -regains -momentum -focus -shifts -smaller -high -quality -projects? (accessed 17 August 2023).

23. Among others, see 'China's Global Development Initiative is not the BRI reborn', *Nikkei Asia*, https:// asia .nikkei .com/ Opinion/ China -s -Global -Development -Initiative -is -not -the -BRI -reborn; 'Global Civilization Initiative proposed by Xi "provides hope to heal the world in turbulence"', *Global Times*, https:// www.globaltimes.cn/page/202303/1287427.shtml; 第一观察 | 总书记首提全球文明倡议意义非凡--时政--人民网 [The mention of the Global Civilisation Initiative by the General Secretary is extraordinarily significant], *People China*, http://politics.people.com.cn/n1/2023/0318/c1001-32646804.html; 'How China can multilateralize the Belt and Road', *Asia Times*, https:// asiatimes .com/ 2023/03/how-china-can-multilateralize-the-belt-and-road/; 'The Global Security Initiative concept paper', https:// www .fmprc .gov .cn/ eng/ wjbxw/ 202302/ t20230221_11028348.html (all links in this note accessed 23 March 2023).

24. David Arase, 'The relationship between BRI and FOIP' webinar, Taipei School of Economics and Political Science, 11 May 2023.

25. Van Jackson, *Pacific power paradox: American statecraft and the fate of the Asian peace* (New Haven, CT: Yale University Press, 2023). When asked about his view on 'American primacy' as a policy, Assistant Secretary of State for East Asian and Pacific Affairs Daniel J. Kritenbrink said that he had not heard of this term in the corridor of power in Washington, DC, at the New Zealand Institute of International Affairs conference, Auckland, 8 June 2023.

26. Susan Thornton, 'How the West should meet the China challenge', Ellsworth Memorial Lecture, delivered at the 21st Century China Center, School of Global Policy and Strategy, University of California at San Diego, 16 March 2023.

27. 'How Saudi Arabia and UAE are positioning themselves for power', *Financial Times*, reprinted in *Weekend Herald*, Auckland, 26 August 2023, p. C6.

28. What if geo-developmentalism is shifting from China's initiation to other countries taking similar initiatives? Although this phenomenon is gradually evolving and the question is a bit hypothetical at present, it is worth pondering for the sake of clarifying the definition. At the moment and in the foreseeable future, China is expected to dominate in initiating huge infrastructure projects around the world, with an increasing number of partnership countries and host countries working with it. Other countries are also beginning to initiate their own programmes and projects, for one reason or another, but they are small in number and in scale in comparison. Even if these projects are initiated, up, and running, it can be seen that they have been stimulated by China's BRI, which means that China is still instrumental in spreading geo-developmentalism. I am grateful to one of my

book manuscript reviewers at Edward Elgar Publishing for pointing this out to me.

29. See: https://www.who.int/director-general/speeches/detail/who-director-general-s-speech-at-the-paris-peace-forum-panel-act-a-covid-19-vaccines-tests-and-therapies-the-global-public-good-solution---12-november-2020 (accessed 10 August 2022).

30. See: https://blogs.imf.org/2022/01/12/support-for-africas-vaccine-production-is-good-for-the-world/ (accessed 25 July 2022).

31. See: https://www.ethicsandinternationalaffairs.org/journal/after-liberal-hegemony-the-advent-of-a-multiplex-world-order (accessed 18 August 2023).

Bibliography

BOOKS, JOURNAL ARTICLES, AND REPORTS

Alves, Ana Cristina D., 'BRI and global development praxis: is a paradigm shift eminent?', in Joseph Chinyong Liow, Liu Hong, and Gong Xue (eds), *Research handbook on the Belt and Road Initiative* (Cheltenham, UK, and Northampton, MA, USA, 2022), pp. 81–83.

Benatar, Solomon, and Gillian Brock (eds), *Global health: ethical challenges*, 2nd ed (Cambridge: Cambridge University Press, 2021).

Cao, Jiahan, 'Toward a Health Silk Road: China's proposal for global health cooperation', *China Quarterly of International Strategic Studies*, Singapore, Vol. 6, No. 1 (2020), pp. 19–35.

Cao, Zhang et al., 'The legislative approach and system improvement of China's compulsory licensing for drug patents', *Drug Design, Development and Therapy*, Dovepress, No. 15 (2021), p. 3717.

Chan, Gerald, Pak K. Lee, and Chan Lai-Ha, *China engages global governance: a new world order in the making?* (London and New York: Routledge, 2012).

Chan, Gerald, *China's digital Silk Road: setting standards, powering growth* (Cheltenham, UK, and Northampton, MA, USA: Edward Elgar Publishing, 2022).

Chan, Gerald, *China's maritime Silk Road: advancing global development?* (Cheltenham, UK, and Northampton, MA, USA: Edward Elgar Publishing, 2020).

Chan, Gerald, *Understanding China's new diplomacy: Silk Roads and bullet trains* (Cheltenham, UK, and Northampton, MA, USA: Edward Elgar Publishing, 2018).

Chang, Kyung-Sup, *The logics of compressed modernity* (Cambridge: Polity, 2022).

'China's global vaccine gambit', *Nikkei Asia*, part 1: production, politics and propaganda, 12 October 2021, https://asia.nikkei.com/static/vdata/infographics/chinavaccine-1/ ; part 2: pharmacy of the world, 23 December 2021, https://asia.nikkei.com/static/vdata/infographics/chinavaccine-2/; part 3: the great medicines migration, 5 April 2022, https://asia.nikkei.com/static/vdata/infographics/chinavaccine-3/.

'China's international development cooperation in the new era', White Paper, Information Office, State Council, People's Republic of China, January 2021, https://english.www.gov.cn/archive/whitepaper/202101/10/content_WS5ffa6bbbc6d0f7 2576943922.html.

'Coronavirus disease (COVID-19) pandemic', WHO, https://www.who.int/europe/emergencies/situations/covid-19.

'Development of China's public health as an essential element of human rights', White Paper, Information Office, State Council, PRC, September 2017.

Garlick, Jeremy, *The impact of China's Belt and Road Initiative: from Asia to Europe* (London: Routledge, 2019).

Gurgula, Olga, 'Compulsory licensing vs. the IP waiver: what is the best way to end the COVID-19 pandemic?', South Centre, Geneva, policy brief, No. 104

(October 2021), https://www.southcentre.int/wp-content/uploads/2021/10/PB104_Compulsory-licensing-vs.-the-IP-waiver_EN-2.pdf.

Hale, Zachary A., 'Patently unfair: the tensions between human rights and international property protection', *Arkansas Journal of Social Change and Public Service*, Vol. 7, No. 1 (4 April 2018), https://ualr.edu/socialchange/2018/04/04/patently-unfair/.

Jiang, Yonghong, *Zhongguo yimiao bainian, 1919–2019* [*One hundred years of Chinese vaccines, 1919–2019*] (Hong Kong: Kaifang shudian, 2021).

'Joint communique of the leaders roundtable of the second Belt and Road Forum for International Cooperation', Beijing, 27 April 2019, http://www.xinhuanet.com/english/2019-04/27/c_138016073.htm.

'Keywords to understand the Global Development Initiative', Academy of Contemporary China and World Studies, July 2022, http://keywords.china.org.cn/2022-07/24/content_78338443.html.

Lee, Seow Ting, 'Vaccine diplomacy: nation branding and China's COVID-19 soft power play', 6 July 2021, *Springer Nature Limited*, https://doi.org/10.1057/s41254-021-00224-4.

Li, Mingjiang, 'The BRI: fuelling strategic rivalry between China and the United States', in Joseph Chinyong Liow, Hong Liu, and Gong Xue (eds), *Research handbook of the Belt and Road Initiative* (Cheltenham, UK, and Northampton, MA, USA: Edward Elgar Publishing, 2021), pp. 416–25.

Lin, Shaun, Naoko Shimazu, and James D. Sidaway, 'Theorising from the Belt and Road Initiative', *Asia Pacific Viewpoint*, Wellington, New Zealand, Vol. 62, No. 3 (December 2021), pp. 261–9.

Malkin, Anton, 'The made in China challenge to US structural power: industrial policy, intellectual property and multilateral corporations', *Review of International Political Economy*, 2020, https://doi.org/10.1080/09692290.2020.1824930.

Meng, Qingyun, (ed.), *Zhongguo zhongyiyao fazhan wushinian (1949–1999) [Fifty years of development of Chinese medicine (1949–1999)]* (Zhengzhou: Henan Medical University Press, 1999).

Ordu, Aloysius Uche, *Foresight Africa: top priorities for the continent in 2022* (Africa Growth Initiative at Brookings, 2022), Chapter 2: Public health: ensuring equal access and self-sufficiency, pp. 26–45.

Ou, Jiezheng, *Dang zhongyi yushang xiyi* [*When Chinese medicine meets Western medicine*], rev edn (Hong Kong: Joint Publishing [H.K.] Co., Ltd., 2023).

Seligsohn, Deborah, 'The key role of multilateral coordination in the U.S.–China health relationship', in Lucas Myers (ed.), *Essays on China and U.S. policy* (Washington, DC: Wilson Center, 2022), pp. 194–221.

Shadlen, Kenneth C., Bhaven N. Sampat, and Amy Kapczynski, 'Patents, trade and medicines: past, present and future', *Review of International Political Economy*, Vol. 27, No. 1 (2020), pp. 75–97.

The industrial map of China pharmaceuticals, 2006–2007 (in Chinese) (Beijing: Social Sciences Academic Press, 2006)

Tu, Zhuxi, *'Zhongguo ji lu' yu pingxing shijie: Covid-19 yiqing shidai de Zhongguo shijiao guancha* [*'China's Road' and a parallel world: Chinese perspectives and observations in the Covid-19 era*] (Hong Kong: Joint Publishing (H.K.) Co., Ltd., 2022).

'Vaccine manufacturing in Africa', DCVMN member briefing – presentation document, UK Aid, 17 March 2021.

'Vision and actions on jointly building Silk Road economic belt and 21st-century maritime Silk Road', State Council, People's Republic of China, March 2015, https://www.fmprc.gov.cn/eng/topics_665678/2015zt/xjpcxbayzlt2015nnh/201503/t20150328_705553.html.

'Vision for maritime cooperation under the Belt and Road Initiative', State Council, People's Republic of China, June 2017, https://english.www.gov.cn/archive/publications/2017/06/20/content_281475691873460.htm.

Whittaker, Hugh D., et al., *Compressed development: time and timing in economic and social* development (Oxford: Oxford University Press, 2020).

WHO global report on traditional and complementary medicine 2019 (Geneva: World Health Organisation, 2019), p. 8.

World intellectual property indicators 2019 (Geneva: World Intellectual Property Organization, 2019),

World intellectual property indicators 2020 (Geneva: WIPO, 2020),

Xi, Jinping, 'Work together to build the Silk Road economic belt and the 21st century maritime Silk Road', speech at the opening ceremony of the Belt and Road Forum for International Cooperation, Beijing, 14 May 2017, http://2017.beltandroadforum.org/english/n100/2018/0306/c25-1038.html.

Zhongguo yidaiyilu nianjian [Yearbook of China's Belt and Road Initiative] (Beijing: China Commerce and Trade Press, 2019).

NEWSPAPERS AND MAGAZINES

21st Century Business Herald, China
BBC World Service
China Daily
Hong Kong Economic Journal
Huanqiu shibao [Global Times], China
Ming bao, Hong Kong
New York Times
Nikkei Asian Review, Tokyo
Quishi [Seeking Truth]
Renmin ribao [People's Daily]
South China Morning Post, Hong Kong
Weekend Herald, Auckland
Yazhou zhoukan [Asiaweek], Hong Kong

WEB SOURCES

'Belt and Road Initiative', *Xinhua*, https://www.xinhuanet.com/silkroad/english/mobile.htm.

Belt and Road Portal, https://www.yidaiyilu.gov.cn/.

Belt and Road Research Platform, Leiden Asia Centre, https://www.beltroadresearch.com/.

Bridge Consulting (Beijing) Co., Ltd., https://bridgebeijing.com/about/.

China Africa Research Institute, SAIS, Johns Hopkins University, http://www.sais-cari.org/.

China Connects, International Institute for Strategic Studies, IISS China Connects.

Chongyang Institute for Financial Studies, Renmin University of China, https://www
.rdcy.org.

Clingendael: Netherlands Institute of International Relations, Silk Road headlines, Silk
Road Headlines Archive, Clingendael, https://www.clingendael.org/publication/silk
-road-headlines-archive.

Mercator Institute for China Studies, https://merics.org/en.

National Development and Reform Commission, China, http://en.ndrc.gov.cn/.

National Health Commission, China, http://en.nhc.gov.cn/publications.html.

Reconnecting Asia, Center for Strategic and International Studies, https://
reconnectingasia.csis.org/.

Silk Road Fund, https://www.silkroadfund.com.cn.

Appendix: a chronology of ten years of developments of the BRI, 2013–23

2013 September	Xi Jinping proposes the building of the Silk Road Economic Belt in Kazakhstan
2013 October	Xi Jinping proposes the building of the 21st-Century Maritime Silk Road in Indonesia
2013 December	The 3rd Plenum of the 18th Chinese Communist Party Congress commits to develop the BRI
2014 February	Xi and Putin of Russia reach an agreement on linking the BRI with the Eurasian rail line
2014 March	Li Keqiang stresses the development of the BRI in the government working report
2014 April	Li stresses the importance of the BRI in an opening speech at Bo'ao Forum for Asia
2014 May	China–Kazakhstan joint logistics terminal opens in Lianyuangang in Jiangsu province, the first official project in the Silk Road Economic Belt
2014 November	Xi announces at the APEC summit that China will contribute US$40 billion to set up the Silk Road Fund
2014 November	The first annual World Internet Conference, or Wuzhen Summit, held in eastern China
2015 March	Fifty-seven countries join the Asian Infrastructure Investment Bank as founding members
2015 March	The Chinese government publishes a policy paper on 'Vision and Action on Jointly Building Silk Road Economic Belt and 21st-Century Maritime Silk Road'
2015 April	The SRF's first major investment: China–Pakistan Economic Corridor
2015 May	'Made in China 2025' starts: a strategic plan to nurture 20 advanced technologies within ten years with an investment of US$300 billion
2015 September	Xi announces the establishment of the South–South Cooperation Assistance Fund at the UN General Assembly. The initial instalment amounts to US$2 billion
2015 October	The Silk Road Think Tank Network (SiLKS) established with 43 founding members and partners from 27 countries
2016 June	The AIIB extends its first batch of loans to Bangladesh, Indonesia, Pakistan, and Tajikistan

2017 January	China and the WHO sign a memorandum of understanding on the BRI, focusing on global health
2017 May	Belt and Road Forum for International Cooperation held in Beijing; 'Beijing Communiqué of the Belt and Road Health Cooperation and Health Silk Road' signed by China, WHO, UNAIDS (the Joint United Nations Programme on HIV and AIDS), and 30 countries
2017 June	The Chinese government publishes a policy paper on 'Vision for Maritime Cooperation under the Belt and Road Initiative'
2017 October	The 19th Chinese Communist Party Congress enshrines the BRI in the Party constitution
2018 January	The Chinese government publishes a policy paper on 'China's Arctic Policy'
2018 March	'China Standards 2035' project starts
2018 July	US starts the 'trade war' with China
2019 March	Italy signs a memorandum of understanding on the BRI with China, becoming the first western European country to do so
2019 April	The second Belt and Road Forum for International Cooperation held in Beijing
2019 May	Donald Trump bans Huawei with a national security order
2020 January	The first phase of Sino–US trade agreement signed
2020 January	WHO declares Covid-19 as public health emergency
2020 April	China announces the donation of US$30 million cash to the WHO to combat Covid-19
2020 May	Xi Jinping announces at the World Health Assembly a US$2 billion fund to assist affected nations in their Covid response
2020 July	First Chinese Covid vaccine trial outside of China commences in Brazil
2021 May	Xi pledges to contribute an additional US$3 billion over three years to aid the global response to combat Covid-19
2021 June	Joe Biden announces the Build Back Better World plan at the G7 summit in the UK to counter the BRI
2021 June	'Asia and Pacific High-level Conference on Belt and Road Cooperation' meeting online
2021 September	Xi proposes the Global Development Initiative at the UN General Assembly
2022 February	Russia invades Ukraine
2022 April	Xi proposes the Global Security Initiative at the Bo'ao Forum for Asia
2022 June	G7 leaders announce the establishment of the Partnership for Global Infrastructure and Investment at a summit in Germany
2023 March	Xi proposes the Global Civilisation Initiative at the Dialogue of World Political Parties
2023 October	Jakarta–Bandung high-speed rail scheduled to start operation
2023 October	The third Belt and Road Forum for International Cooperation scheduled to be held in Beijing, on the occasion of the tenth anniversary of the Belt and Road Initiative

Index